Contents

CRIPPLING A NATION

Health in Apartheid South Africa

AZIZA SEEDAT

idaf

International Defence and Aid Fund for Southern Africa
London April 1984

All photographs are from the photo library of IDAF Research Information and Publications Department. Cover photo by Nancy Durrell-McKenna.

The International Defence and Aid Fund for Southern Africa is a humanitarian organisation which has worked consistently for peaceful and constructive solutions to the problems created by racial oppression in Southern Africa.

It sprang from Christian and humanist opposition to the evils and injustices of apartheid in South Africa. It is dedicated to the achievement of free, democratic, non-racial societies throughout Southern Africa.

The objects of the Fund are:–

   (i)   to aid, defend and rehabilitate the victims of unjust legislation and oppressive and arbitrary procedures,

  (ii)   to support their families and dependents,

 (iii)   to keep the conscience of the world alive to the issues at stake.

In accordance with these three objects, the Fund distributes its humanitarian aid to the victims of racial injustice without any discrimination on grounds of race, colour, religious or political affiliation. The only criterion is that of genuine need.

The Fund runs a comprehensive information service on affairs in Southern Africa. This includes visual documentation. It produces a regular news bulletin 'FOCUS' on Political Repression in Southern Africa, and publishes pamphlets and books on all aspects of life in Southern Africa.

The Fund prides itself on the strict accuracy of all its information.

ISBN No. 0 904759 54 7

List of Tables

Preface

South Africa is the only country in the world where racial discrimination is enshrined in the constitution. Apartheid is a system of oppression and exploitation of the black majority in South Africa as a source of cheap and expendable labour. They have been put into this position by armed force and by numerous laws which have denied them the shares of the land and its wealth which are their birthright.

Any discussion of health in South Africa, therefore, must take place in a political and economic context. As a consequence of apartheid policies, health care provision for blacks is grossly inadequate. This is reflected in the statistics of mortality rates and the incidence of disease which are the direct result of the poverty, deprivation and the harsh conditions of life allotted to the black majority.

The aim of this book is to present the facts about the health of the South African people. In the following chapters, various aspects of health care and health under apartheid are considered.

It is hoped that the hypocrisy of the 'separate but equal' argument of the protagonists of the apartheid system will be revealed. 'Health' under apartheid for the majority of the population is a story of suffering, illness and disease. A free, readily available and non-discriminatory health service will only be achieved with the destruction of the apartheid system and the establishment of a non-racial South Africa where health for all the country's people is a basic right and priority.

For the guidance of the reader, **Chapter 1** comprises a statistical overview of the health of the South African people and the health policies of the regime. **Chapter 2** is intended as an introduction to the apartheid system as such and briefly describes its political, economic and social implications for the black majority. **Chapter 3** examines the incidence and underlying causes of malnutrition and infant mortality among black South Africans, while **Chapter 4** surveys the varying incidence of the most common infectious diseases in South Africa.

Chapter 5 moves to the realm of the workplace to look at the various health hazards and risks which confront South African workers, and the adequacy or otherwise of industrial health legislation. **Chapter 6** describes conditions in state and private mental hospitals and reviews the incidence of psychiatric illness and disorder among black and white South Africans.

7

Chapters 7 and **8**, covering health and welfare services, and health workers, respectively, describe the state's response to ill-health, its prevention and cure, and the variable access to health facilities enjoyed by black and white South Africans. **Chapter 9** introduces the reader to the ethical and political questions raised for health workers by the maltreatment of political detainees, and to the ongoing campaign for the international isolation of the South African medical profession.

Note: The four main population groups in South Africa, according to the official classification system, are African (21.0 million, or 72.7 per cent of the population), white (4.5 million, 15.5 per cent), Coloured (2.9 million, 9.0 per cent) and Indian (0.8 million, 2.8 per cent). These figures are for 1980, and are based on the official census, together with estimates for the 'independent' bantustans.

1. Introduction — Some Statistics

A country's basic health services are judged on two main criteria: the infant mortality rate and the life expectancy of its population.

A study of the health situation in South Africa reveals two distinct patterns of diseases for black and white people respectively. White South Africa has a pattern similar to that found in the developed countries: a low infant mortality rate (14.9 per 1,000 live births in 1978 — similar to that in Britain)[1] and a long life expectancy (64.5 years for white males and 72.3 for females for the period 1969-71).[2] (The infant mortality rate measures the number of babies who die before their first birthday, not including those still-born.)

Black South Africans, particularly Africans, have a health pattern similar to that of underdeveloped countries: high infant mortality rates and low life expectancies. It has been estimated that in some rural parts of South Africa, between 30 and 50 per cent of children die before their fifth birthday. In May 1983, the infant mortality rate among Africans in Worcester, Cape Province, was reported to be 550 per 1,000.[3]

Official figures of life expectancy for Africans have not been available since 1945-47 when the life expectancy for an African male was 36 years and that for a female, 37. At the time, this was 20 years less than the life expectancy of whites.[4] Life expectancy figures have not been available since then because it has not been compulsory for Africans to register births or deaths, and authoritative demographic figures cannot be compiled.

The latest available official estimates give Africans life expectancies of 51.2 for males and 58.9 for females, for the period 1965-70,[5] and an infant mortality rate of 100-110 per 1,000 live births for the year 1974.[6]

It has been estimated that at least 50,000 deaths among black people annually are not registered. These occur mainly in the rural areas. Birth statistics for Africans are not published by the government.[7] One consequence of the 'independence' of the bantustans is that it becomes even more difficult to obtain statistics to cover them, while figures for 'South Africa' (i.e. excluding the 'independent' bantustans) conceal the true incidence of disease.

Official life expectancies for the years 1969-71 for Coloureds are 48.8 years for males and 56.1 for females, and for Indians, 59.3 for males and 63.9 for females.[8] *(See also Table IV)*.

In stark contrast to the experience of black people, white South Africans suffer from the diseases of affluence familiar to the western industrialised world. For these, they enjoy some of the highest standards of medical care in the world. The mortality rate from coronary heart disease amongst whites was by 1982 the highest in the world, and two-and-a-half times higher than in the United States. Heart disease has caused South Africa to be dubbed the 'coronary capital' of the world.[9]

TABLE I: The main causes of death in South Africa, 1976.

According to figures compiled by two South African medical researchers, the 10 most important causes of death among the four main population groups in 1976 were as follows:–

Order of importance	White	Indian	Coloured	African
1	Ischaemic heart diseases	Ischaemic heart diseases	Enteritis & other diarrhoeal diseases	Pneumonia (excluding viral pneumonia)
2	Cerebrovascular diseases	Cerebrovascular diseases	Pneumonia (excluding viral pneumonia)	Enteritis & other diarrhoeal diseases
3	Pneumonia (excluding viral pneumonia)	Pneumonia (excluding viral pneumonia)	Cerebrovascular diseases	Homicide & wilful injury by others
4	Motor vehicle accidents	Hypertension	Ischaemic heart diseases	Cerebrovascular diseases
5	Bronchitis, emphysema & asthma	Motor vehicle accidents	Homicide & wilful injury by others	Tuberculosis of the respiratory system
6	Malignant neo-plasms of the trachea, bronchus & lung	Enteritis & other diarrhoeal diseases	Immaturity (not specified)	Immaturity (not specified)
7	Senility (without psychosis)	Immaturity (not specified)	Tuberculosis of the respiratory system	Motor vehicle accidents
8	Venous thrombosis & embolism	Bronchitis, emphysema & asthma	Motor vehicle accidents	Anoxic & hypoxic conditions
9	Diseases of the arterioles & capillaries	Diabetes mellitus	Bronchitis, emphysema & asthma	Malignant neo-plasm of the oesophagus
10	Suicide & self-inflicted injury	Cirrhosis of the liver	Hypertension	Measles

Source: H. C. J. van Rensburg & A. Mans, *Profile of Disease and Health Care in South Africa,* Academica, Pretoria/Cape Town/Johannesburg, 1982, p.78, Table 22. The figures are for 1976, and are compiled from various official statistical sources.

Among the black population, particularly the Coloured and African groups, unnatural deaths through homicide and violence take a major toll of adult lives. Diseases of the respiratory system, notably tuberculosis, pneumonia, enteritis and other diarrhoeal diseases, and heart disease of a kind thought to be related to malnutrition, are as or even more important. Hypertension (high blood pressure) is the second most common cause of heart failure amongst African adults. It is found particularly among the urban population and affects both men and women, often killing both in their 30s or 40s. This severe form of hypertension is extremely rare in rural Africans. It has been suggested that stress in the urban areas, under apartheid conditions, may be a factor.[10]

In 1978, typhoid fever was forty-eight times more common among blacks than whites,[11] while in 1971 deaths from diarrhoea were one hundred times more common among black children than whites in Cape Town.[12]

The figures for the most common causes of death (*see Table I*) illustrate the violent character of South African society. Such violence has its roots in the poverty and frustration of the conditions of life for the black population, and the militaristic and repressive character of the South African state. Among Coloureds and Africans, 'homicide and wilful injury by others' is the most important cause of unnatural death, and, respectively, the fifth and third most important cause of death overall. Among whites and Indians, motor vehicle accidents constitute the main cause of unnatural deaths, with suicide rising to second place as a cause of unnatural death, and tenth as a cause of death overall, among whites.

TABLE II: Reported causes of murder and homicide, 1979.

Murder	—	white by black	112
	—	white by white	133
	—	black by black	6,495
	—	black by white	99
	—	infanticide (all groups)	74
Culpable homicide	—	white by black	20
	—	white by white	84
	—	black by black	3,461
	—	black by white	135

Source: Annual Report of the Commissioner of the South African Police for the period 1 July 1978 to 30 June 1979.

In 1974-5 South Africa spent 3.6 per cent of its Gross National Product (GNP) on health, a decline from 4.2 per cent in 1959-60.[13] This proportion is lower than for some countries with lower per capita incomes.

11

The health service structure in South Africa is geared towards the disease patterns of whites with the bulk of resources spent on expensive high technology diagnostic and curative services. Ninety-eight per cent of the medical budget is spent on curative services 'usually supplied to an urban elite at high cost'.[14] It has been estimated that only two per cent of expenditure on health care in South Africa is devoted to preventative medicine.[15]

It is also interesting to note that the white population in South Africa has a higher proportion of patients suffering from renal failure being treated by dialysis and/or transplant treatment than in almost any other country in the world. The figure of 107 per million is exceeded only by Israel, the U.S.A. and Switzerland, but is almost double the European average of 57 and the British rate of 62 per million. In contrast the figure for black South Africans is four per million.[16]

By the same token expensive heart transplants are performed for the few while Soweto has the highest incidence of rheumatic heart disease in the world, a disease which could be eradicated by improving living conditions. South Africa spends at least R24,000 a day on heart operations for rheumatic heart disease, rather than on preventative measures. (This emphasis on curative rather than preventative measures is also illustrated in the amount of money spent on heart transplant operations — a procedure pioneered in South Africa.)

Moreover, 21 per cent of total health expenditure in South Africa goes on drug sales, 50 per cent on non-ethical and 50 per cent on ethical drugs.[17] (Non-ethical drugs have not necessarily been approved for safety purposes and do not require a prescription; ethical drugs require a doctor's prescription). In fact it has been estimated that 25 to 30 per cent of hospitalised patients suffer complications as a result of adverse drug reactions due to polypharmacy. (Polypharmacy is the practice of treating patients with more than one drug, and usually many, at a time). The South African pharmaceutical industry spends four times as much on promotion as on research, and the system is directed at the needs of white patients rather than black.

Discriminatory attitudes are evident in family planning services, which are largely concerned with controlling the size of the black population. White fears of being 'swamped' by a numerically much larger black population are evident in exhortations to whites to increase the size of their families. In 1976 state spending on family planning was increased to R5.3 million, the Minister of Health justifying the amount by saying 'one does not want to curtail funds in this connection because this is also a matter with a bearing on our survival, viz. when we allow the population to increase unhindered.'[18] In November 1981, the Director-General of the Department of Health, Welfare and Pensions, Dr. Johann de Beer, warned that sterilisation and abortion might have to be made compulsory unless 'certain ethnic groups' accepted family planning measures. In evidence to the Science Committee of the President's Council, he pointed out that while the white and Indian birth rates both currently stood at 16 per 1,000, the Coloured birth rate was 26 per 1,000 and the African 35 per 1,000.[19]

Medical education, too, tends to focus on the problems suffered by the better-off. In a survey published in 1978 of fourth year white medical students at the University of Cape Town only six per cent said they were planning to practise community medicine when they qualified. Furthermore, when asked how well the medical school equipped them for each of the following, the students placed 'a doctor in a teaching hospital' first, followed by 'medical care for people in a Westernised society', 'specialisation', 'research and teaching' and 'an urban general practitioner', in that order. Community health came *ninth* on the list and medical care in a developing African country came *tenth*.[20]

On the other hand, black doctors reported that they saw their main problems as lying in the socio-economic conditions of the blacks in the country. They expressed mounting frustration at the sheer grinding poverty of the black people of South Africa. Over a third of black medical students felt that their medical education did not provide them with adequate training to deal with these problems. A significant proportion wished to have a course of social and preventative medicine reintroduced into the syllabus.[21]

Because of the high standard of medical care for its white citizens, South Africa is often regarded as a country with a good health service. The now defunct South African Department of Information (in the late 1970s the centre of a huge scandal involving dubious undercover activities and the secret use of vast amounts of state funds) published many books and glossy magazines presenting a favourable picture of South Africa, including its health services.

One of the Department's main themes was the high standard of health care in South Africa and this was one of its most powerful weapons in its bid to sell South Africa's image abroad. The world's first heart transplant, performed at Groote Schuur Hospital in Cape Town in 1968, gave the South African government some of its best propaganda in years.

The impact of South African propaganda should not be underestimated. It certainly is effective, as illustrated by the fact that many doctors from abroad, including Britain, still emigrate to South Africa with a view to gaining more experience and expertise. Medical conferences in South Africa are still attended by many delegates from other countries and South African experts are still invited to address major conferences the world over. This contributes to a general picture of South Africa as a country in the forefront of medicine.

However, if this propaganda is carefully scrutinised, it will be revealed to be a mixture of truths, half-truths and some outright lies. Photographs are carefully posed and selected. For example in 1977 the Department of Information published a pamphlet entitled *The Health of the People* including a full page colour picture of an African patient on renal dialysis at Baragwanath Hospital — suggesting that such treatment was readily available for blacks.

Another distortion is the statement that 'all the health services are available to all the inhabitants of the Republic irrespective of race, colour or religion'[22] or the statement by a South African diplomat on BBC television that 'we have only a few cases of malnutrition'.[23]

Furthermore, South African propaganda never compares facilities available for blacks in South Africa with those for whites in South Africa, but instead compares facilities available for blacks in South Africa with those for blacks elsewhere in Africa, and in so doing actually juggles with statistics to deceive the reader. For example, in *Health and Healing*, another pamphlet issued in 1969 by the Department of Information in Pretoria, figures are given for the ratio of the number of doctors per population in South Africa, but these are figures for *all* population groups combined. If the figures of the ratio of serving doctors to population are given for the different groups separately, it will be found that there are fewer serving black doctors per head of the black population than in any of the other African states mentioned, with the exception of Burundi, Chad, Rwanda, Upper Volta and Dahomey — countries much poorer than South Africa *(see also Chapter 8)*.

Figures for infant mortality quoted tend to be the very lowest figures. For example, *Health and Healing* has the figure of 68 per 1,000 for Soweto in 1968, but not mentioned is the figure of 269 per 1,000 for the previous year in Port Elizabeth. Other unreliable information is contained in the 1970 issue of *Report from South Africa*, another official publication. This cites a figure of 23,000 for the number of 'Bantu nurses'. Two years later, in April 1972, the figure was only 11,000 according to the same official magazine.

The truth of the matter is that at the present time South Africa's health services remain dominated and controlled by whites and deeply permeated by apartheid. The majority of the people are shut out from any real part in the political decisions shaping health care in South Africa and cannot participate in decisions about the distribution of health resources or the design, development and future direction of services.

The achievement of an adequate health service available to all South Africans, irrespective of class or colour, will never be realised until the apartheid system is destroyed. South Africa is a highly industrialised and wealthy country, but the ill-health of its black population, suffering from the diseases of poverty, malnutrition and deprivation, serves as a damning indictment of the apartheid regime.

2. The Bantustans, Migrant Labour and Poverty

This chapter looks in more detail at the political, economic and social conditions imposed by apartheid on the majority of South Africa's population, the black Africans.

The Land Act and bantustan policy

In South Africa 71 per cent of the population has been allocated only 13 per cent of the land. This was the result of the *Native Land Act* of 1913 which prohibited Africans from gaining any legal rights to any land outside their 'traditional' areas. It allocated barely more than eight per cent of the land to blacks and reserved the rest for exclusive white ownership. The area of the black reserves was increased to between 12 and 13 per cent by the *Native Land and Trust Act* of 1936.

The political pressure for the passing of these Acts came almost entirely from those who wished to ensure a steady and cheap supply of labour. The only way that South Africa's rulers could force people to accept low wages in the white-owned mines, farms and factories of South Africa was to destroy their self-sufficiency and alternative forms of livelihood.

By the late nineteenth century white farmers were complaining that the blacks were 'rich enough' not to have to work for whites and that they were undercutting white farmers and buying up all the land.[1]

Blacks were therefore obliged through the passing of the Glen Grey Bill in 1894 to pay taxes. As Cecil Rhodes said at the time, 'We want to get hold of these young men and make them go out to work, and the only way to do this is to compel them to pay a certain labour tax . . . It must be brought home to them that in the future nine-tenths of them will have to spend their lives in daily labour, in physical work, in manual labour.[2]

The 13 per cent of the land allocated to Africans under the Land Acts is in scattered parcels, largely in the Transvaal, Orange Free State and Natal, apart from the Ciskei and Transkei, both in the Cape Province. These areas were originally known as Native Reserves; in 1959 they were renamed 'bantu homelands' and quickly dubbed 'bantustans'. Today the official terminology is 'black homelands', 'black states', or 'national states'. There are a total of 10 such 'homelands', four of which have been declared 'independent'.

The apartheid government often tries to project a rosy picture of the bantustans. One official publication explains that 'the Bantu homelands contain more than sufficient land for the growing of the quantity of grain and raising the amount of animal protein, fruit and vegetables required by the entire Bantu population of South Africa . . . the anomaly is that a large part of South Africa's best areas in the most favourable climatic belts is in the hands of the least competent farmers or more accurately, in the hands of men who do not farm at all.'[3]

Some of the land allotted to Africans in the 'best areas' has suffered from drought for long periods. Soil erosion is rife and there is extreme overcrowding.

The average population densities in the bantustans are much higher than in other parts of South Africa. The preliminary results of the 1980 official census indicated population densities for the non-'independent' bantustans ranging from 53.7 persons per square kilometre in KaNgwane to 254.2 persons per square kilometre in QwaQwa, total area a mere 620 sq. km. and in essence little more than a sprawling rural slum. In the 'independent' bantustans of Transkei, Bophuthatswana and Venda, population estimates compiled for 1980 by the Bureau for Economic Research indicated densities of 53.1, 30.0 and 42.6 persons per sq. km. respectively.[4] The population density for the whole of South Africa, excluding Transkei, Bophuthatswana and Venda, was 21.9 persons per sq. km. according to the 1980 census.[5]

Unofficial estimates of the bantustan populations suggest even higher densities. The *de facto* populations have been increasing very rapidly — and continue to do so — as a result of the South African government's apartheid policies of forced removal and relocation of black people. Between 1970 and 1980 the population of KaNgwane, in particular, increased by 204 per cent, that of KwaNdebele by 415 per cent and QwaQwa, 515 per cent.[6]

Because of the gross overcrowding in the bantustans there is simply not enough land to cultivate. Food and money are both in short supply. Figures compiled for 1980 by the Bureau for Economic Research (BENSO) showed that over 5.2 million Africans living in the bantustans had no measurable income.[7] A survey of the 'independent' bantustans (Transkei, Bophuthatswana, Venda and Ciskei) in 1981 revealed average annual *per capita* incomes ranging from R230 (in Venda) to R453 (in Ciskei). Between 39 and 52 per cent of cash income was spent on food.[8]

The problems of the bantustan areas are aggravated by the fact that the population is unbalanced, with a high proportion of the young, the old and the disabled — those who are not required as labour by the apartheid economy.

17

It has been estimated that one third to one half of the adult male population in the bantustans is absent at any one time, contributing to the low level of farming. Many women are also forced to seek work elsewhere to support their families. In general they are excluded from seeking work in the industrial areas of South Africa and the majority work as domestics or in agriculture.

There are very few job opportunities in the bantustans and, in general, very little economic activity takes place within their borders. Over the two decades from 1960 to 1980, only 75,000 jobs were created within the bantustans through development corporation investment, with a further 75,000 created in 'border industries'.[9] In 1980, only 13 per cent of the income of the bantustans was generated inside their boundaries.[10]

Migrant labour

Africans are resident in the white areas only as long as their labour is required, and must return to the bantustans when their contracts terminate or they become unemployed. They are considered 'temporary sojourners' in white South Africa. The 1922 Stallard Commission stated that the African 'should only be allowed to enter the urban areas, which are essentially the white man's creation, when he is willing to enter and to minister to the needs of the white man, and should depart therefrom when he ceases so to minister'.[11] This is still the policy which applies today.

Removals may involve the eviction of whole settlements in rural areas designated as 'white' and the removal of individual African men and 'superfluous appendages' (women and children) from the cities by endorsing them out under the influx control laws. The *Black Urban Areas Act*, Section 10, prohibits any African from remaining in an urban area longer than 72 hours unless s/he can prove that s/he has permission to live and work there and has resided in the area continuously since birth, or has worked continuously for an employer for not less than 10 years. The migrant worker is contracted to work in the city for 12 monthly periods with one month in the bantustans. He or she therefore never qualifies for permanent residence. The *Bantu Law Amendment Act* of May 1964 placed a total ban on the further entry of African females into the urban areas, other than on a visitor's permit, for a specified and restricted period. Following the recommendations of the Riekert Commission in 1979, this ban was partially relaxed, while at the same time tighter restrictions were placed on other workers attempting to move to the cities.

The movement of Africans is closely controlled by means of the pass laws or influx control regulations. Every African over the age of 16 is required to carry a pass book at all times, his or her fingerprints on the pass book are filed in a central register in Pretoria, and the records computerised and connected to all the main cities in the country. If the passbook cannot be produced on demand, the person is almost certain to be arrested.

The figures for arrest and prosecution under the pass laws are very high. Between 1948 and 1981 at least 12.5 million people were arrested or prosecuted. Conviction leads to a fine or imprisonment or removal to the bantustans. In 1979, those sentenced under the pass laws constituted one third of all convicted prisoners in South Africa's jails.[12]

The bantustans serve as reservoirs of cheap black labour for white South Africa and dumping grounds for the elderly, the infirm, women and children. The forced removals of people into the bantustans, the historical expropriation of African lands in the last century and the present extension of the migrant labour system have made the majority of Africans dependent on money incomes for their existence. The African population has in fact not been self-sufficient for the past 60 years and if the bantustans were to become viable in the sense of providing jobs for all their citizens, the cheap labour that tills the fields, mines the gold and fills the factories of South Africa would be lost.

The migrant worker's family is prohibited from joining him during the months of his employment, except on short visits, and the result is inevitable demoralisation and disruption of family life. In the urban areas outside the bantustans there is a high ratio of males to females while in the rural areas the opposite applies.

The influx control system is particularly firmly enforced in the Western Cape area because this has been declared a 'Coloured preference area' where Africans may not be employed if any other population group is available. As a result two thirds of all males employed in Cape Town industries in 1969 were migrant workers, with their families living away in the bantustans. In the mid-1970s, the rigour with which the influx control laws were applied was interrupted and as a result many came to Cape Town to join their menfolk. As no new family housing was officially provided these families began to build their own homes in squatter settlements such as Crossroads. Here, they were always at the mercy of apartheid officials who could demolish their homes and split the families up again.

It is admitted that black labour is needed in the white areas. But, as former Prime Minister John Vorster said, 'the fact that they work for us can never entitle them to claim political rights. Not now, not in the future. It makes no difference whether they are here with any degree of permanency or not...'[13] This statement, made in 1968, is still fundamental to apartheid policy today.

TABLE III: Comparative monthly earnings, 1981.

Sector	Average monthly earnings (rand)			
	White	Coloured	Indian	African
Mining	1,197	361	567	201
Manufacturing	1,074	297	336	255
Electricity	1,046	425	—	256
Construction	1,069	328	506	193
Trade and accommodation services	648	231	339	165
Transport and communications	945	246	498	242
Finance and insurance	864	417	533	305
Government and services	786	307	575	208
Total	890	293	413	216

Source: SAIRR, 1982, p.64, citing the National Manpower Commission Report for 1981.

Poverty in South Africa

The Gross National Product (GNP) of South Africa is one of the highest in Africa and among the top 30 in the world, but the wealth is very unevenly distributed. Whites, comprising 15 per cent of the population, received 64 per cent of national income in 1977, while Africans (73.5 per cent of the population) received 26 per cent.[14] On average, a white worker earns more than four times the monthly wage of an African (*see Table III*).

Figures for average *per capita* incomes show even greater discrepancies: for the year 1974-75, *per capita* personal incomes for the main population groups were white R2,534, Indian R584, Coloured R496 and Africans R237 — less than one tenth those of whites.[15]

The comparison of *per capita* African incomes in South Africa with those elsewhere in Africa is also instructive, particularly as white South Africans are fond of claiming that 'their' Africans are better off than Africans anywhere else. For 1980, the South African Institute of Race Relations calculated that the real *per capita* Gross National Product (GNP) in the bantustans (excluding KwaNdebele) ranged from R120 (Gazankulu) to R314 (Bophuthatswana). The *per capita* GNP in Nigeria (1978) was US$600 (c.R726 at late 1983 exchange rates); it was US$620 (R750) in Botswana (1978), US$440 (R532) in Angola (1979), US$240 (R290) in Mozambique and in Tanzania (1978), US$300 (R363) in Lesotho (1978) and US$380 (R460) in Kenya (1978), to cite a few examples.[16]

20

The standard of living of Africans in South Africa is in general very low. The majority live in poverty because of inadequate wages and widespread unemployment. Agriculture and services employ the largest fractions of the African labour force — officially 18.6 and 22.6 per cent respectively in 1980.[17] There is no minimum wage for African farm workers in South Africa. In 1952 the average African farm labourer's income was assessed at just over £3 a month and there are figures to indicate that in real terms this average wage stayed almost constant between the discovery of minerals in South Africa (1870s and 1880s) and the end of the Second World War.[18] The agricultural census of 1976 estimated average monthly cash wages for regular farm employees as R31.95 with rations valued at R9 provided.[19] Official figures given in parliament in 1981 indicated that African farm workers could still be earning as little as R32 a month including the food provided by employers — cash wages alone were as low as R23 a month. A government commission was told in 1982 that some farm workers were earning R10 a month.[20] Because of influx control laws farm workers cannot find work elsewhere.

The system that controls African workers functions to preserve cheap labour on the farms. The Labour Bureau classifies a person into one of several categories of employment; once classified, the worker cannot change (except to mine or farm work) and, in particular, he cannot escape from farm work. This system ensures that there is no competition in wages. Despite the fact that wage rates for Africans in manufacturing industry are considerably higher than those in farming and better than those in mining, the farms and mines are never short of labour. Africans in urban areas unemployed for more than four months (not necessarily consecutive) in any year may be arrested and sent to work in farming areas.

In the mining industry the ratio of white to black incomes actually widened from 9:1 in 1911 to nearly 20:1 in 1971.[21] Although the ratio fell to just under 6:1 in 1981, the gap between average white and African monthly wages increased from R360 to R996.[22] African wages have in general been increased over the last decade but they never approach white wages and in most years have been effectively eroded by inflation.

The Poverty Datum Line (PDL) is an estimate of the lowest income average families need for existence. A somewhat more generous estimate, sometimes called the Minimum Effective Level (MEL) or Household Effective Level (HEL), allows for spending on education, furniture, cooking utensils, leisure and modest savings as well as the basic necessities of the PDL. It is usually about 50 per cent higher than the PDL.

The monetary level of these poverty lines varies from month to month and city to city. But at any given time, a large proportion of African families in South Africa, even in the relatively affluent cities, is living below the breadline. Thus in 1976 a market research survey showed that two thirds of all African households had less than R80 a month on which to live, 25.4 per cent had between R80 and R149 and only 11 per cent had more than R150. Nearly a quarter had less than R20.[23]

This was at a time when it was estimated that a family of five in Soweto needed R129 a month to survive. These figures were confirmed by the Institute of Planning Research at the University of Port Elizabeth which in 1976 showed that in all but one employment sector average African earnings were below the PDL.[24]

A number of surveys of average African household incomes have indicated that these incomes actually declined by 12.4 per cent in real terms between 1976 and 1980.[25] A university-sponsored survey of 837 African families carried out during 1982 in three Port Elizabeth townships revealed that the average monthly household income was R252, compared to the required Household Effective Level of R297. The average monthly earnings of employed household heads were R172, with 50 per cent falling into the R120 to R285 income range and 25 per cent earning less than R120 a month.[26]

Another survey of 800 African families in various parts of South Africa in March 1982, by the Markinor African Syndicate, produced an overall average household income of R351 a month.[27]

The percentage of each main population group living in poverty was calculated in 1978 as follows: white two per cent, Coloured 50 per cent, Indian (on the East Rand) 20 per cent and (in Durban) 50-60 per cent, and African between 60 and 70 per cent.[28] The situation in the rural areas for Coloured and African families in particular tends to be worse. In Nqutu in the KwaZulu bantustan, for example, the average monthly income was reported to be R20 in 1980.[29]

The claim that black wages in South Africa are rising, and with them the standard of living of Africans, must be measured against the high figures for unemployment. The exact extent is difficult to ascertain as comprehensive figures are not kept, but in 1978 it was estimated that over two million African workers were unemployed and that the total was increasing by 470 a day.[30]

Private local surveys have found unemployment rates of 19 per cent among Africans in Cape Town, 24 per cent in Pretoria and 28 per cent in Johannesburg and the Reef. Estimates for rural bantustan areas range up to 42 per cent in Limehill, KwaZulu.[31] Underemployment is common with Africans working seasonally in the farms and plantations, or obtaining jobs on short contracts for a few months before being laid off.

The official figures published by the South African government indicate that unemployment has declined since the beginning of the 1980s. In September 1981, a total of 134,459 people (5,767 white, 6,970 Coloured, 2,484 Indian and 119,238 African) were registered as unemployed at employment offices. This was the lowest figure since 1976.[32]

Regional estimates by the government for June 1981 showed 10.6 per cent unemployment among Africans in the cities (Coloured 4.3 per cent), 6.0 per cent among Africans in towns (Coloured 4.3 per cent), 3.6 per cent on farms (Coloured 2.8 per cent) and 9.9 per cent in the bantustans. Overall the figures were African 7.8 per cent and Coloured 4.1 per cent.[33]

Academics and other experts have criticised the government's figures as underestimates of the true position. A seminar at the University of the Witwatersrand in October 1982 was told that about 2.5 million people or 24 per cent of the labour force were unemployed. Other estimates cited by the South African Institute of Race Relations place the unemployment figure at between 1.5 and 3 million.[34]

Families without incomes or land to cultivate cannot hope to provide nutritious food or sanitary surroundings for themselves and their children. The economic, social and political status of Africans under apartheid ensures that the vast majority live in conditions of great poverty and deprivation. The effect that these conditions have on their health and well-being is analysed in the following chapters.

3. Malnutrition and Infant Mortality

Malnutrition is the single biggest killer of black children in South Africa. One of the myths propagated by the South African government is that although poverty is a factor, 'ignorance', 'bad eating habits', 'superstition' and 'taboos' are largely to blame. The truth of the matter is that in the face of grinding poverty it is simply impossible to obtain enough of the right kind of food for adequate nutrition. One study concluded, for example, that the 'mother's educational level was irrelevant to the child's nutrition, but rather that there was severe and almost universal poverty'.[1] Taboos have also been investigated and have been found to have no significance.[2]

The main diseases of malnutrition are kwashiorkor and marasmus. Kwashiorkor has been described as the most severe nutritional disease known.[3] It characteristically follows weaning and results from a diet grossly deficient in milk and other high protein foods. There may be an associated deficiency of vitamins and calories. Marasmus is the childhood equivalent of starvation. It has its onset in the first year of life when supplementary feeding is not provided. It is due to a severe deficiency of calories together with some deficiencies in protein.

Incidence of malnutrition

In *Health and Healing*, a South African government information pamphlet (*op. cit., Chapter 1*), it is stated that 'kwashiorkor . . . was proclaimed notifiable in South Africa so that a clear picture of its incidence and distribution might be obtained.' The figures that are given for the incidence of kwashiorkor amongst Africans from 1963 (15,477) to 1967 (9,765) suggest that it has declined.[4]

Kwashiorkor in fact ceased to be a notifiable disease in 1967. The last official figures published for that year were: whites seven cases, Indians 12, Coloureds 1,046 and Africans 9,765 cases.[5] When questioned as to whether kwashiorkor would again be declared a notifiable disease, the Minister replied that it would not.[6] The reason given was that the notifications of kwashiorkor were 'unreliable' due to the different interpretations of the diagnostic criteria in this field.

Medical and nursing staff throughout the black hospitals in South Africa, however, both urban and rural, report incidences of malnutrition of almost epidemic proportions. Their findings are confirmed by other

24

sources. A commission of inquiry into conditions in the Ciskei bantustan, for example, reported that kwashiorkor and marasmus, the two most important nutritional deficiency disorders, were endemic. Their incidence was 27 per cent and 4.5 per cent respectively in the age group six to 23 months.[7]

A survey conducted by the South African Institute of Race Relations in 1978 revealed that 50 per cent of all two to three year old children in the Ciskei were malnourished. Urban Ciskeian children had an incidence of kwashiorkor and/or marasmus of one in ten, while for rural children the incidence was one in six.[8] A clinic in the Northern Cape, where 200 children attended daily, reported in 1980 that 'nearly all' were suffering from malnutrition.[9]

Staff at a Bophuthatswana hospital serving a population of 100,000 people claimed in 1980 that as many as 40 per cent of deaths were due to malnutrition. They estimated that 50,000 children would probably die directly or indirectly of malnutrition in the rural areas of South Africa and that a further 100,000 children's lives were at risk.[10]

In 1979 it was reported that 8,000 children per year died in hospitals in Natal and Kwazulu. Two thousand of these casualties occurred at the major teaching hospital in Durban, King Edward VIII. The deaths were directly or indirectly attributable to malnutrition.[11]

Such news items are not uncommon in South Africa. The problem is long-standing and unchanging. During the 1980s, however, the situation has been aggravated by the worst drought that South Africa has experienced for two centuries — a drought that has not only affected South Africa but neighbouring countries as well. In April 1983 the head of the Department of Paediatrics at the University of Natal, Professor Allie Moosa, claimed that South Africa's current death toll from malnutrition stood at 30,000 a year, or three to four an hour — the vast majority of the victims being children.[12] His appeal to the South African government to take preventative action, however, met with little positive response. The Minister of Health, Dr. C. V. van der Merwe, said that responsibility for the high toll of dying children should be shared by those people who continued to 'multiply uncontrollably'.[13] The deputy Director of Health said that statistics showed that a total of 4,061 people died from 'dietary conditions' in 1978, of whom 3,171 were African, 403 Coloured, 105 Indian and 382 white.[14]

Infant mortality

A survey in 1979 demonstrated the following:

- Mortality rates for both African and Coloured children aged one to four years were 13 times as high as for whites.

- The majority of deaths occurred in children under five years of age.
- Deaths below one year were six times higher among Africans and Coloureds than among whites.[15]

TABLE IV: Percentages of deaths according to age, 1970.

Age category	White Pop(%)	White Deaths(%)	Coloured Pop(%)	Coloured Deaths(%)	African* Pop(%)	African* Deaths(%)
0 – 4	11	7	17	49	16	55
5 – 24	38	4	48	6	46	7
25 – 44	26	8	22	11	23	10
45 – 64	18	30	10	16	11	16
65+	7	52	3	18	4	12
Totals	100	100	100	100	100	100

*The figures for the African group are those in selected magisterial districts.

Source: SAMJ, Vol. 55, 1979, p.801; cited in H. C. J. van Rensburg & A. Mans, *Profile of Disease and Health Care in South Africa,* Academica, Pretoria/Cape Town/Johannesburg, 1982, p.21.

TABLE V: Infant mortality rates in various urban centres.

City	Year	Deaths per 1,000 live births White	Coloured	Indian	African
Port Elizabeth	1970	—	—	—	330.00
Johannesburg	1970	20.00	—	—	95.00
Grahamstown	1970	—	—	—	188.00
Bloemfontein	1972	—	—	—	170.00
East London	1972	—	—	—	107.00
Cape Town	1973	—	—	—	63.00
Cape Town	1981	9.40	18.80	20.40	34.60
Pretoria	1980	10.08	53.48	11.98	53.13

Sources: Medical Officer of Health Reports; SAIRR, 1982, p.528.

The South African government does not itself publish national figures for infant mortality rates among Africans. The only figures available, other than estimates, are those compiled by Medical Officers of Health in the main urban areas. These indicate infant mortality rates ranging up to over 300 deaths per 1,000 live births in certain areas (*see Tables IV and V*). The latest available government estimate for the whole country (excluding the 'independent' bantustans) is 100 — 110 per 1,000 live births, for the year 1974.[16]

26

TABLE VI: Comparative infant mortality rates, by country.

Country	Year	Deaths per 1,000 live births
Australia	1980	10.7
Canada	1981	9.6
Denmark	1979	8.8
Finland	1979	7.7
Greece	1979	18.7
Iceland	1979	5.4
New Zealand	1980	13.0
Norway	1980	8.1
Poland	1980	21.2
Portugal	1979	26.0
Romania	1979	31.6
Switzerland	1979	8.5
UK-England & Wales	1980	12.0
UK-Scotland	1980	12.1
USSR	1974	27.7

Note: The 1984 report of the United Nations Children's Fund (UNICEF), published in December 1983, identified three countries — Upper Volta, Afghanistan and Sierra Leone — as still having infant mortality rates higher than 200 per 1,000 live births. Sweden, Finland and Japan had the lowest average figures with only seven infant deaths per 1,000 births; Britain, Singapore and Ireland had 11 deaths per 1,000 births. South Africa, with 90 infant deaths per 1,000 births, had one of the highest rates in relation to national wealth, the report found. In 1981, the year to which the figures related, the *per capita* Gross National Product (GNP) was calculated as R2,300. Kenya, GNP R460 a head, had an infant mortality rate of 80 per 1,000, and Uganda, GNP R240, a rate of 100 per 1,000 (*Tel.* 8.12.83; *Star,* 19.12.83).

Source: Demographic Yearbook 1980, information provided by Office of Population Censuses and Surveys, London, December 1983.

National infant mortality rates for the other population groups in 1978 were: white 14.9 per 1,000, Coloured 80.6 per 1,000 and Indian 25.3 per 1,000.[17] (*Table VI shows figures for other countries.*)

The high infant mortality rates among black South Africans occur in a country that, by comparison with the great majority of independent African countries, has a booming economy and prides itself on being a major exporter of food. In the early 1960s thousands of tons of surplus fruit and bananas were dumped to rot, 4,000 lbs of butter were exported to Britain at a loss, and 23 million bags of maize were in storage awaiting export. In 1976 the Dairy Board reported that farmers in Bloemfontein were pouring more than 10,000 litres of milk down the drain daily.[18] In 1971, under the headline 'Too much Food — South Africa's Dilemma', a newspaper report revealed that surplus milk powder was being fed to animals and that eggs were exported at a loss.[19] Similarly, in 1980, it was reported that record maize harvests had been achieved but large quantities were being exported at a loss. The result was an increase in domestic prices, notably the prices of bread and mealie meal — the staple diet of blacks in South Africa.[20]

Vitamin deficiency diseases

Vitamin deficiencies are very common in South Africa as a result of malnutrition in children and adults. Pellagra, rickets and beri beri are all examples of deficiency diseases. Eight to 20 per cent of black children in South Africa have been reported to be suffering from rickets, a disease due to Vitamin D deficiency.[21] Pellagra, due to a deficiency in nicotinamide, is by far the commonest vitamin deficiency disease in African adults. According to Department of Health estimates there were 100,000 cases in 1979.[22] Thirty three per cent of the adult population in a district of the Ciskei were found to be suffering from pellagra in 1980 while 50 per cent of children were victims of marasmus.[23] Whites very rarely suffer from pellagra except in a mild form and usually among vagrants.

Beri beri is the result of thiamine deficiency and is thought to be directly responsible for a form of heart failure. In Johannesburg about one fifth of all cases of 'African cardiomyopathy' were found to be thiamine deficient, and at Stellenbosch the figures were similar.[24] It is generally accepted that this condition is associated with chronic malnutrition and/or the excessive intake of alcohol.

Cardiomyopathy is becoming increasingly frequent amongst the male migrant workers living in single-sex hostels in South Africa's big cities. The majority of patients with this disease are found to come from these hostels. The workers exist on a poor diet (often consisting of a 'coke and bun') and drink excessive amounts of 'Bantu beer' which is extracted from maize. Professor Seftel of the University of the Witwatersrand said at his inaugural lecture in 1973 that alcoholism and chronic malnutrition resulted from these unnatural living conditions and led to fatal heart disease.[25] The authorities encourage drinking by building beer halls next to the hostels, and a large percentage of the income spent on Soweto and other black townships comes from the profit made on these premises by the Administration Board. Drink has become the focal point of social life in the absence of families, homes and recreational facilities, and one of the few forms of pleasure amidst the grim living quarters and after a harsh working day. Pellagra is also common amongst migrant workers.

Rather than doing away with the whole system which creates these hostels, the Department of Health now adds Vitamin B to beer, and nicotinamide and riboflavin to maize meal, to prevent pellagra. Similarly, to combat malnutrition and also with South Africa's international image in mind, a scheme of distributing subsidised skimmed milk to pre-school children was devised during the 1960s. The scheme was ineffectual, partly due to inadequate facilities for distribution. Despite an admission to this effect from the Department of Health in 1974,[26] *Health and Healing* (*op. cit.*) claimed that '. . . skimmed milk powder . . . is subsidised and distributed extensively . . .'. Since 1974 skimmed milk powder has been replaced or supplemented by PVM, a concentrate of protein, vitamins and minerals.

Effects of malnutrition

Malnutrition contributes both directly and indirectly to the mortality rate. One of the major causes of death is the infection to which a malnourished child is particularly susceptible. The most common of such infections is gastro-enteritis. Figures from the Department of Statistics from the years 1968-71 inclusive showed that deaths from gastro-enteritis amongst Coloured children totalled 23,752, i.e. an average of 5,938 deaths per year.[27]

The incidence of gastro-enteritis appears to be rising. There were more infant deaths from this cause in the first five months of 1976 than during the whole of 1975 according to the then Professor of Paediatrics at the Red Cross Hospital in Cape Town.[28]

In 1982, a total of 50,000 children were estimated to die each year in South Africa from malnutrition and malnutrition-related diseases, with gastro-enteritis as the biggest killer[29] (*see also Table I*).

Other effects of malnutrition include stunted growth. The *South African Medical Journal*, for example, reported that:

- In 1977 in Soweto 66.4 per cent of children between the ages of two and five weighed less than normal.
- Of the same group 29.1 per cent were shorter than normal and in the case of 20.1 per cent of the children their weight/height ratio showed that they were malnourished. (The weight/height ratio was normal in less than 80 per cent of the cases, i.e.).
- In a study in Muldersdrift in 1976 of children aged between one and six years 27.6 per cent were found to be underweight and 22.8 per cent were shorter than normal.
- Among rural children under the age of seven, 47.3 per cent in the Transvaal were underweight. Of the urban children 40.3 per cent were underweight.
- 55.6 per cent of rural nursery school children aged between one and six years were underweight.[30]

Studies of better-off African and Coloured children have proved beyond doubt that their growth attainment becomes comparable to western standards as the economic status of the family improves. The authors of one such study came to the conclusion that growth retardation was 'strikingly' associated with poverty.[31]

The mental effects of malnutrition are also well documented. Medical researchers have established that malnutrition during the first two years of life has harmful consequences for brain growth and it appears that the resulting deficiencies in intellectual function are permanent. Marasmus particularly affects brain growth, ocurring as it does at a younger age and therefore having the maximum effect on brain growth.

The high rate of malnutrition among black children in South Africa, and the rising incidence of marasmus in particular, have devastating implications for future generations of black South Africans.

4. Infectious Diseases

Tuberculosis

Infectious diseases which have been practically eradicated in developed parts of the world, are still a serious problem among South Africa's black population. By far the most widespread of these is tuberculosis (TB), accounting for over 80 per cent of all notifiable diseases in South Africa[1] (*see Tables VII and VIII*). Apart from kwashiorkor, TB is the single most important cause of severe morbidity and death for the African population. Ten people are estimated to die *every day* from TB in South Africa,[2] a figure which in any developed country would be regarded as totally unacceptable.

Official figures released by the Department of Health underestimate the true incidence of TB. The Department calculates the actual number of cases to be three times the number of official notifications, but the South African National Tuberculosis Association (SANTA) has found the incidence to be five to ten times higher. The recorded incidence of TB has lain between 42 and 45,000 officially notified cases in recent years, suggesting that there may be as many as 150,000 or more actively diseased or infected people in the country at any time.[3] The head of the community health department at Medunsa (Medical University of South Africa) stated in 1982 that the incidence of TB was 150 to 200 for every 100,000 people; of these 82 per cent were African. He said that about 110,000 people had active TB while about 10 million had it in dormant form.[4]

Tuberculosis is rife in the bantustans. In 1970 the medical journal *The Lancet* reported that TB was present in 20 per cent of babies under six months and that the majority of adults in the Transkei showed evidence of TB.[5] Over 27 per cent of notified cases of TB in 1981 were in the bantustans (*see Table VII*).

While the incidence of TB has halved amongst whites since the beginning of the 1970s it has increased by more than 40 per cent amongst blacks. In 1980 a total of 2,050 deaths were officially attributed to TB.[6] Although preventive BCG immunisation of new-born babies became mandatory in 1973, the inoculation service has tended not to reach those born outside clinics or hospitals, particularly in outlying rural districts.[7]

The cost of TB in terms both of human suffering amongst black South Africans and of the health budget is immeasurable. In spite of the introduction of outpatient treatment in recent years, in 1978 there were still

TABLE VII: Incidence of tuberculosis by region, 1981-82.

	1981	Notified cases of TB 1982 (January to September)
Cape East	5,861	4,153
Cape West	8,651	6,681
Cape North	2,138	1,709
Natal	4,749	3,107
Orange Free State	3,255	2,146
Transvaal South	12,040	8,716
Transvaal North	1,019	805
Sub-Total	37,713	27,317
Ciskei	2,007	1,156
Gazankulu	89	21
KwaZulu	5,001	2,611
Lebowa	766	250
QwaQwa	102	177
KaNgwane	501	390
Bophuthatswana	2,001	1,357
Transkei	3,712	1,573
Venda	121	74
Sub-Total	14,300	7,609
Total	52,013	34,926

Source: SAIRR, 1982, pp.526-7, citing figures given by the South African Department of Health.

TABLE VIII: Incidence of tuberculosis by population group, 1979.

Group	Notified cases	%
White	606	1.35
Coloured	8,326	18.50
Indian	673	1.50
African	35,094	77.99
Other	299	0.66
Total	44,998	100.00

Note: Official information about the number of TB cases on each population group is available only for 1977 and 1979.

Source: SAIRR, 1980, p.559.

23,000 hospital beds provided for TB patients in state, SANTA, local authority and private institutions. Annual costs for hospitalisation alone at the time were estimated at R25 million.[8] By 1981 this had dropped to a total of 10,678 beds. The 1982-83 budget allocated R48,072,700 to combat TB, of which R31,223,300 was for hospitalisation.[9] The cost of drug therapy for TB in South Africa is amongst the highest in the world. The drug Rifampican, for example, which is given two to three times a week, costs R1.80 a day. Elsewhere in Africa it costs the equivalent of 20 cents.[10] In recent years, Rifampican has been in chronic under-supply in South Africa. To be effective, drug treatment for TB out-patients needs to be sustained over a considerable period of time in a supportive environment — conditions which are unlikely to be met for black South Africans.

Tuberculosis has been shown to decrease in incidence with a rising standard of living, better nutrition and improved housing, but in South Africa no attempt is made to tackle the problem from this angle. Instead, expensive measures are taken in the urban areas to treat the disease out of concern that whites might catch it through contact. Typical attitudes were revealed during the 1979 debate on the health vote in the House of Assembly when Dr. A. L. Boraine referred to reports 'which indicate that a great number of patients suffering from tuberculosis are disobeying and disregarding doctors' and hospitals' orders and are thus a menace to society at large'. The Minister of Agriculture interjected 'They must drink more milk instead of Coca Cola!'[11]

Gastro-intestinal infections

In combination with malnutrition and infections such as TB and pneumonia, gastro-enteritis accounts for the majority of deaths in black South African children.[12] It is a non-notifiable disease. At King Edward VIII Hospital in Durban, gastro-enteritis, dysentery and typhoid accounted for 13 per cent of admissions over 16 years.[13] This did not include non-specific gastro-enteritis, which occurs as a complicating factor in malnutrition and other diseases.

Typhoid

Typhoid is also widespread amongst the black population. In 1980, 17 out of every 100,000 South Africans were diagnosed as having typhoid.[14] Overall, more than 3,000 cases of typhoid are reported annually.[15] Official figures for 1979 and 1980 were 3,784 and 3,721 reported cases, respectively.[16] Periodic outbreaks of typhoid, which is closely associated with poor hygiene, lack of clean water and inadequate garbage removal and sewerage, occur in the black 'resettlement' areas and squatter camps.

TABLE IX: Incidence of certain notifiable diseases, 1981.

	Bantustans	Rest of South Africa	Total
Diphtheria	28	29	57
Malaria	975	1,335	2,310
Measles	5,970	8,135	14,005
Meningococcal infection	99	983	1,082
Poliomyelitis	62	64	126
Tetanus	183	148	331
Typhoid	1,866	1,857	3,723
Viral hepatitis	239	1,549	1,788

Source: SAIRR, 1982, p.531, citing SA Department of Health figures.

TABLE X: The 12 most important notifiable diseases, 1976.

Diseases, in order of importance by total number of notifications	Notifications Total	Rate per 100,000	Notifications per 100,000 in main population groups White	Indian	Coloured	African
1. Tuberculosis	56,304	218.70	17.4	71.0	295.0	262.0
2. Typhoid fever	3,254	12.68	2.3	3.4	2.8	16.8
3. Infective hepatitis	1,795	6.97	16.2	30.6	6.9	3.8
4. Malaria	1,747	6.79	3.2	0.8	0.04	6.1
5. Meningococcal infection	1,240	4.82	3.3	0.9	14.0	4.1
6. Trachoma	818	3.18	0.0	0.0	0.0	4.5
7. Scarlet fever	689	2.68	14.4	0.3	1.0	0.2
8. Diphtheria	343	1.33	0.2	0.1	1.0	1.7
9. Poliomyelitis	328	1.27	0.1	0.3	2.5	1.4
10. Tetanus	326	1.27	0.0	0.4	0.9	1.7
11. Encephalitis	299	1.16	4.2	0.9	0.4	0.5
12. Leprosy	146	0.57	0.1	0.1	0.3	0.7

Source: H. C. J. van Rensburg & A. Mans, op. cit., p.96, citing S.A. Department of Health figures.

Cholera

In recent years South Africans have been alarmed by several outbreaks of cholera. The disease, first identified in Nelspruit in the northern Transvaal in late 1980, had by the end of 1982 officially killed 234 people in the course of two epidemics. (The figure excluded Bophuthatswana and Transkei).[17]

The first epidemic, in 1980-81, officially accounted for 22 deaths, while 1,372 people were treated.[18] Other sources reported that 4,000 victims were infected, the majority of them black people living in squalid conditions in resettlement areas in the bantustans.[19] In the Bophuthatswana bantustan people were being infected from the Apies River whose water they were obliged to use out of financial necessity. 'Safe' water cost about 15 cents a litre in the bantustan and the inhabitants could simply not afford it. Rather than trying to provide an alternative and freely available supply of clean fresh water, the Bophuthatswana government passed an act making it unlawful for villagers to draw water from the infected Apies River.

Alarm mounted when it was discovered that the disease had spread from the bantustans in northern Transvaal to Natal, the Orange Free State and even Soweto, with cholera strains being found in the sewage of Johannesburg.[20]

During the second, even more serious epidemic, 212 people died and 62,852 clinically confirmed cases were treated, according to official figures. The majority of the latter, 50,503, were in KwaZulu and Natal.[21]

Cases of cholera continued to be reported into 1983, and in February, the Minister of Health and Welfare stated that it had accounted for 69 deaths over the period February 1982-January 1983 inclusive. With the exception of two victims in Natal, who may have been Coloured, all those who died were African. Once again, the figures excluded the 'independent' bantustans.[22]

The official figures issued by the Department of Health and Welfare were disputed as being too low, and there was also criticism of the way in which the government had gone about combating the disease. Dr. Liz Thomson of the University of Cape Town, for example, said that the state's health education campaign had largely consisted of distributing posters and pamphlets to people who were usually illiterate. She said that people were being told to boil their water when they did not have enough fuel, and to keep human wastes away from water supplies when they had no sanitation. In this way, the state had 'shifted the blame' for cholera away from the socio-economic conditions of apartheid and on to the people themselves.[23]

In March 1983, the Minister of Health and Welfare in the KwaZulu bantustan, Dr. Dennis Madido, said that the disease had now become endemic in KwaZulu. He compared cholera to a crocodile, which would come out of the water to feed and then go back in, but would never go away.[24]

There have been outbreaks of cholera in South Africa before. In 1974, an outbreak in the gold mines was traced to the faecal contamination of drinking water consumed during acclimatisation exercises. Recruits were infected after they had arrived at the mines clear of the disease.[25]

Other diseases

Measles is a serious disease amongst black children because of underlying malnutrition. It is often fatal, and has become the second most common notifiable disease in South Africa with a total of just over 14,000 recorded cases in 1981 (*see Table IX*). In 1982, it was said to be claiming 11 lives a day.[26] In Port Elizabeth alone, 54 children died of measles during 1982, and 145 during the first four and a half months of 1983.[27] The nationwide immunisation campaign does not effectively extend into the bantustans and much of the rural areas.

Malaria is endemic in certain sub-tropical areas along South Africa's northern and eastern borders. Its incidence has fluctuated, but in general has tended to increase since the late 1960s, in line with worldwide trends. A particularly high figure of notifications, 3,271, was recorded in 1977, a year of heavy rainfall in the susceptible areas.[28]

The incidence of **venereal disease** in South Africa is increasing. Amongst the black population, the migrant labour system and the consequent social disruption are major factors in its occurrence. About 8,000 cases of gonorrhoea and more than 3,000 of syphilis were treated during the year to mid-1981 at clinics in Alexandra, Rosslyn and Badplaas in the Transvaal.[29] In Cape Town in 1972 the incidence of venereal disease per 1,000 population was white, 1.6 and black, 22.4. In the Cape Flats area, a desolate ghetto area for Coloured people in the Cape, the incidence of venereal disease was estimated to be as high as 40 to 60 per cent. Pregnant women tested at a clinic in Graaf Reinet in the Eastern Cape showed positive Wasserman Reactions (a test for the presence of syphilis) in 12 to 17 per cent of cases.[30]

It has been estimated that 10 per cent of new born babies in Soweto have a positive Wasserman Reaction. The number of cases of congenital syphilis at King Edward VIII Hospital in Durban rose from 14 in 1960 to 68 in 1973 and 22 per cent of the babies affected died.[31]

The incidence of **rheumatic heart disease** amongst Africans has already been referred to (*see Chapter 1*). The disease occurs in conjunction with poor living conditions and has been largely eradicated in industrialised countries.

In 1982, a survey of 1,150 schoolchildren in Hout Bay, Cape Town, indicated that seven out of every 1,000 black South African children under the age of 15 had rheumatic heart disease. Seven of the children examined had rheumatic fever and 60 had cardiac murmurs. Dr. P. E. Bundred, senior lecturer in community health at the University of Cape Town, said that 50 per cent of cases went unnoticed in the community. Five per cent of the children surveyed would need heart operations at some stage, and would probably have their life spans cut down to no more than 20 years.[32]

Dr. Bundred pointed out that the disease could be prevented by a single dose of intra-muscular penicillin each month. However, in contrast to the United States, where every school had a school nurse, in Soweto there was only one state school nurse for 1.5 million people.[33]

Trachoma, the greatest single cause of blindness in developing countries, is endemic in certain areas of South Africa, especially the northern Transvaal, along the Limpopo river, the Lebowa bantustan and the Louis Trichardt area. It is a disease of poor hygiene, spread by flies, or among family members using the same towel or face cloth. In some villages it is responsible for a blindness rate of 0.5 per cent while in parts of Gazankulu over 80 per cent of the people are affected.[34]

In March 1982 a **polio** epidemic broke out in the north-eastern Transvaal and the Gazankulu and Lebowa bantustans. By August of that year a total of 286 cases had been confirmed and 45 people had died — compared with 126 reported cases in the whole of the country in 1981.[35] There was considerable criticism of the health authorities during the epidemic for their failure to ensure that immunisation measures were effective and that they reached all children.[36] The great majority of polio victims are black and the disease has been almost eradicated amongst whites.

Another disease associated with conditions of poor sanitation and general deprivation, also found in South Africa, is **bubonic plague.** Plague is spread to humans via fleas from infected rats. During 1982 the settlement of Coega in the eastern Cape was placed in quarantine for just over a week after an outbreak of the disease, and one person later died.[37] Over the Cape Province as a whole, 18 cases of bubonic plague were reported that year,[38] and the disease was said to be endemic in parts of the Cape, the Orange Free State, the Transvaal and South African-occupied Namibia.[39] **Leprosy** is another disease which still occurs in South Africa. In 1983, 152 people were being treated for the disease.[40]

In recent years, as the regime's master-plan of forced removals has continued, the true incidence of particular diseases has been masked by the creation of 'independent' bantustans. Some diseases have made dramatic reappearances after gaps of several years. The available figures, inadequate as they are in many instances, show that the black population, and particularly Africans, suffers most from infectious diseases, almost all of which could be prevented by improved standards of living and better health services.

5. Occupational Health

South Africa's cheap labour economy and the resultant superprofits have attracted many foreign investors. Considerable publicity has been given in recent years to the 'code of conduct' approach to foreign investment, whereby transnational corporations are asked to observe codes of behaviour such as that drawn up by the European Economic Community to 'promote racial equality in employment practices'. Few transnationals have implemented the codes fully in practice, however. South African-registered companies (of which the giant Anglo-American Corporation is the best-known example), together with South African state corporations, have even less reason to be swayed by the pressures of international opinion and protest.

Within this context, it comes as no surprise to find the health and safety of the black workforce being accorded low priority in managerial decision-making. This is reflected in the lack of adequate health and safety standards in South African mines, farms and industries. Indeed, it is often cheaper for management to simply replace injured workers than to introduce accident prevention measures. The rising unemployment rate and the fact that the majority of strikes are illegal help to maintain labour 'peace'.

In other countries Factory Acts reflect the struggles of the workers for better working conditions. Wages and the enforcement of healthy working conditions essentially represent costs to management which reduce profits. In South Africa the basic conditions for good industrial health are denied to the majority of workers. In the past, African workers could not form or join trade unions and were denied recognition and bargaining rights. In 1979 the law was changed to allow some African unions, mainly in the manufacturing sector, to be registered, but even these find there are many obstacles to effective union activity. Unions which do not toe the government line are harassed and their leaders detained and in some cases severely tortured. Dr. Neil Aggett, who was found hanged in detention in February 1982, was a prominent trade union activist.

Even for legally recognised unions the enforcement of industrial health standards has been explicitly prevented by the use of secrecy provisions in the various acts and by the exclusion from the Workmen's Compensation Act of civil actions against an employer. Such factors help to explain the high incidence of industrial and occupational diseases found within the South African economy.

TABLE XI: Industrial accidents, 1974-76.

Year	Total accidents	Permanent disablements	Fatalities	Man hours lost
1974	359,758	32,019	2,284	30,191,054
1975	355,615	31,819	2,232	29,926,332
1976	340,063	33,752	2,546	32,534,762

Note: The Commissioner's Report notes that the lower figure given for total accidents in 1976 is a result of the decrease in employment in that year.

Source: Annual reports of the Workmen's Compensation Commissioner.

Industrial accidents

The annual reports of the Workmen's Compensation Commissioner from 1974 to 1976 show that on average there were some 350,000 reported accidents each year in factories, leaving an average of more than 2,300 workers dead and 32,000 permanently disabled.[1] In 1982 the Minister of Manpower gave the figure of 309,085 accidents for the year 1978. In 1979 there were 299,523 accidents and 3,017,990 man days lost.[2]

The general manager of the National Occupational Safety Association said in 1982 that during the course of that year 31,000 people would be permanently maimed and more than 2,000 killed in industrial accidents. More than 100,000 hands, 50,000 feet and 40,000 eyes would be badly injured. Although the current average of about 309,000 industrial accidents a year represented a decline from the 620,000 average injuries a year in the 1950s, there was no room for complacency, he said.[3] The reported cases are the most serious ones and for the most part also those that result in external injuries. There are no conclusive figures for the incidence of internal injuries or the results of exposure to noxious fumes or dust.

The Second Schedule of the Workmen's Compensation Act notes, as recognised industrial diseases, those due to exposure to toxic substances, for example, chrome ulceration, lead poisoning, dermatitis, phosphorus poisoning and silicosis (fibrosis of the lungs resulting from inhalation of dust). Compensation is available for these diseases, but in reality it is extremely difficult to prove, and even more difficult to locate the causes.

In 1976 a government commission of enquiry into occupational health headed by Justice Erasmus of the Orange Free State reported that '. . . it has regrettably to be stated categorically that, excepting in the mining industry, industrial health not only occupies a secondary position in industry in this country, but that industrialists have put very little time, money and organisation into the prevention of occupational diseases. This applies to prevention of industrial accidents as well'.[4]

The Erasmus Commission found itself 'so hampered' by poor and unreliable statistics and the lack of uniform industrial health standards that it declared that it was 'almost impossible to determine the prevalence and the incidence of occupational disease in South Africa.'[5]

Even so, the little the Commission could ascertain was very revealing. It was found that at least 230,000 workers in industry in South Africa were threatened with industrial deafness. It was doubtful if 10 per cent were supplied with or used ear protectors or had been properly informed of the noise hazards to which they were exposed.[6]

Pollution and poisoning

Since 1972 there has been an alarming increase in the number of **lead poisoning** cases in South Africa. Many industrial enterprises involving the use of lead would probably face closure if international safety standards were applied. Professor I. Webster of the National Institute of Occupational Research said in 1981 that the lead content in the blood of many South African workers who were exposed to the metal was higher than the level considered safe by the World Health Organisation (WHO). 'South Africa is lagging behind in stipulating the dangerous upper limits of lead in the blood,' he said. 'If we were to adopt the standards laid down by the WHO a very large percentage of the workforce would be laid off.' He pointed out that the maximum allowance of lead in the air of a South African factory was 200 micrograms per cubic metre while the generally accepted level in the rest of the world was 150. The effects of lead poisoning included anxiety, hypertension (high blood pressure), psychological changes, anorexia (loss of appetite), irritation, tremor and sleep disturbances.[7]

The Erasmus Commission found that at least 18,000 workers were exposed to **platinosis** (inflammation of the respiratory canal caused by exposure to platinum salts formed during platinum refining). Twenty seven per cent of workers tested in three factories were found to be suffering from platinosis.[8] The Commission was disturbed to find an apparent lack of concern in the **chrome** industry about the physical welfare of workers, particularly the dangers of their contracting rhinitis, bronchogenic carcinoma and perforated nasal septa.[9] A total of 77,132 workers in 715 factories were found to be exposed to **mercury**, where inhalation of fumes and dust can lead to a variety of health problems and illnesses.[10]

In November 1981, the horrifying incidence of **asbestos dust pollution** in South African mines and factories was exposed in a British television programme compiled by a film crew who had visited the town of Prieska in the Northern Cape. A study by a Cape Town industrial health researcher, Dr. Neil White, released at the same time, showed that Prieska and other towns in the region were heavily polluted with lethal blue asbestos dust. Dr. White found that 33 cases of mesothelioma (cancer of the pleural lining of the lungs and abdomen caused by breathing in asbestos dust) had been diagnosed in Prieska in the past 18 months and that more than 30 people had died in the town. A leading local doctor and the superintendent of the hospital said that he had seen about 900 cases of mesothelioma in the past 42 years. Of 1,000 former employees of a single asbestos mine traced by Dr. White, 270 were found to have asbestosis (scarring of the lungs).[11]

The Prieska asbestos mill had in fact been closed a decade before, in 1971. Two uncovered asbestos dumps still stood on the edge of the town, however, while the unoccupied mill site remained heavily polluted. Journalists found that 'the dust lingers in every corner of Prieska, including buildings, vegetable gardens and residential streets'. Children played on the dumps, while recent renovations at a school had exposed a layer of blue asbestos dust five centimetres thick on the roof beams.[12]

Elsewhere in the Cape, where the asbestos mines were still operating, the pollution was even worse. The Granada 'World In Action' documentary screened on British television showed black employees working in plants and mills thickly encrusted with blue asbestos dust, without respiratory protection, and the countryside and watercourses stained blue with dust. Spokesmen for some of the companies concerned, when challenged about the programme, described it as exaggerated and said that safety precautions had been or were being installed. Others were not available for comment.[13]

South Africa is the world's main producer of blue asbestos, which it uses mainly for reinforcing concrete. Blue asbestos is the country's third largest non-metallic mineral export after coal and diamonds. South Africa also produces white asbestos, but it has lagged behind the rest of the world in setting and enforcing asbestos fibre levels in the working environment in mines and factories. South African specialists do not accept that asbestos is as dangerous to health as it is considered to be overseas. In Sweden, for example, asbestos products are totally banned, while in Britain asbestos may only be used with special government permission. In 1982 the International Metalworkers Federation called for a complete ban on all asbestos by 1985.[14]

In 1940, when the South African government first started recording asbestos fibre levels in the mines, up to 120 fibres were measured in one millilitre of air dust. This amounts to extremely severe pollution — the permissible level in the United States has been two fibres per ml since 1976 and the same standard has been set by the European Economic

Community. The South African authorities subsequently set the permissible level at 45 fibres per ml; this was later reduced to 12 fibres per ml, and in 1982, following the media exposure of the scandal, to five fibres per ml.[15] This is still double the standard set by the USA and the EEC.

In April 1981 it was estimated that about 40,000 workers in South Africa were exposed to asbestos.[16] The country has about 30 asbestos mines, located in the Kuruman and Prieska areas of the northern Cape. In 1981 the main companies involved were Rand Mines, the Griqualand Exploration and Finance Company, Gefco (part of the Afrikaner mining group, General Mining), Duicker Exploration (a subsidiary of the British-based Lonrho Corporation) and Everite, an associate of the Swiss-Belgian Externit group. Externit subsequently pulled out of the South African asbestos industry when its interests were taken over by Gefco. The labour force in the asbestos industry is overwhelmingly black and many are migrant workers. Because the latent period for the onset of mesothelioma can be as long as 30 or even 40 years, many affected workers may never come to the notice of the South African Department of Health. Besides those actually working in the mines and mills, others can be affected — families and other relatives of the workers, local residents and others. Black stevedores in Port Elizabeth who handle pressure-packed bags of asbestos for export, for example, can be in serious danger when the bags get torn or punctured by the hooks used in loading, and the air in the ships' holds becomes choked with dust and fibres.[17] The real figure of those exposed to asbestos is thus likely to be much higher than the estimate of 40,000 cited above.

The South African mining companies concerned — particularly Gefco, which consolidated most of the asbestos industry under its control in October 1981 — have responded to publicity by tackling the problem aggressively, encouraging the industrial world to use more rather than less blue asbestos and arguing that the dangers to health, while real, can be controlled. Gefco began to fight the 'killer dust' image by installing safety equipment at its mines and taking the EEC level of two fibres per ml as its own standard. The company claimed that asbestos had been singled out for international criticism for 'political reasons'. During 1981, one third more asbestos was exported from South Africa than in the previous year, a total of 300,000 tons.[18]

The lax standards of occupational safety found in the asbestos industry in South Africa may have been one of the attractions for foreign investors faced with increasingly stringent safety regulations in their own countries as a result of labour and government pressure. The conditions exposed at the end of 1981 would never have been allowed to continue elsewhere. Asked what would happen if Lonrho had tried to operate a plant comparable to its Wandrag asbestos mine and mill near Kuruman, in Britain, a retired senior British factory inspector said that the place would be closed down immediately and a task force despatched by the Factory Inspectorate to decontaminate the whole surrounding area.[19]

With regard to industrial safety in general, the Erasmus Commission concluded that 'virtually nothing is being done in regard to the physical and biological factors that have a deleterious effect on the health of production workers.' The commissioners attributed this poor showing to indifference on the part of industry, apparent in the small number of industrial health staff employed, the failure to use protective equipment, the absence of warning signs and preventive measures, lack of knowledge of the products handled and scant guidance.[20]

A check by the *Cape Times* on the bodies and organisations affected by the Commission found their spokesmen apathetic and in some cases completely ignorant of the Commission and its findings. The Cape Chamber of Industries' spokesman said that he had not read the Report and a spokesman for the Transvaal Chamber of Commerce had 'nothing to say'. The Cape Town Branch of the National Occupational Safety Association found no one who had heard of the Commission.[21]

Industrial health legislation

South Africa's industrial health legislation is of a kind which tends to encourage indifference to health and safety measures on the part of employers.** Industrial accidents and diseases (outside the mining industry perhaps) do not represent a major cost to management because the enforcement of protective measures is left to statutory bodies such as the Workmen's Compensation Commissioner. The Commissioner pays all further costs and medical expenses, including compensation arising out of claims. In fact, management is protected from any claims instituted directly against it by the injured worker by clauses within the Workmen's Compensation Act. A worker may be protected legally against any third party responsible for an accident and where such accidents are the result of negligence by the employer the worker may apply for increased compensation. An employer whose factory seems to be accident-prone may also be forced to pay a higher levy to the Commissioner.

In practice, however, none of these measures has had the desired effect in reducing accidents. The fact remains that there is no way of

---

**Footnote:* During 1983, South Africa's 1944 Factories Act was replaced by a new Machinery and Occupational Safety Act (6/1983). This was criticised by some commentators as imposing undemocratic and divisive health and safety structure onto workers and their organisations (*SALB*, Vol. 8.8 & 9.9, Sept./Oct. 1983).

significantly forcing employers to pay for accidents which are the result of their own negligence and workers have to be content with the highly unsatisfactory compensation paid out by the Commissioner. It should be noted that the allowances are based on a percentage of the wage the worker earns, so that a black worker will tend to receive lower compensation than a white worker for any particular accident or disablement. Furthermore, ignorance of the existence and procedures of the Workmen's Compensation Commissioner on the part of many black workers means that many may never receive the compensation to which they are entitled.

Section 7 of the Workmen's Compensation Act notes that 'No action at law shall lie by the workman . . . against such workman's employer to recover any damages in respect of any such disablement or death.' While employers are protected from damage arising out of their own negligence, the same advantage is not given to the worker. Section 27 of the Act states that '. . . if the accident is attributed to the serious and wilful conduct of the workman, no compensation shall be payable under this Act unless the accident results in serious disablement or the worker dies in consequence leaving a dependant wholly dependent upon him, and the Commissioner or if authorised by the Commissioner, the employer individually liable may further refuse to pay the cost of medical aid or such portion thereof as the Commissioner may determine.' There is thus little incentive in the Act for employers to introduce protective measures for their workers.

TABLE XII: Accidents in the mining industry, 1974-77.

Type of mine	Year							
	1974		1975		1976		1977	
	Dead	Injured	Dead	Injured	Dead	Injured	Dead	Injured
Gold	489	22,494	498	19,236	557	20,728	594	19,973
Diamonds	23	151	13	96	12	86	n/a	n/a
Coal	84	1,616	100	1,608	86	1,781	120	2,061
Other	195	4,346	154	33,670	141	3,588	n/a	n/a
Total	791	28,607	765	54,610	796	26,183	(890)	(25,579)

n/a – figures not available.

Note: A British mining expert claimed at the beginning of 1984 that the death rate in South Africa's coal mines was probably six times higher than in British mines. Dr. Herbert Eisner, former director of the explosives and flame laboratory of the British Health and Safety Executive, said that the statistics compiled by the South African Department of Mineral and Energy Affairs were based on methods of calculation no longer considered reliable by other important mining countries (*T*, 7.2.84).

Source: SALB, March 1979, Vol. 4, Nos. 9-10, p.49.

The drawing up and enforcement of regulations for the physical protection of workers is the responsibility of the Department of Labour. Within the Department is a Factory Inspectorate whose broad mandate is to enforce the Factories, Machinery and Building Workers Act. The Inspectorate, guided by professional groups such as the Council for Scientific and Industrial Research (CSIR) and the National Institute for Research into Occupational Diseases, formulates more specific regulations. However, the detailed rules are not available to the public and access to them depends on the whim of the factory inspector.

It is very difficult, in consequence, for a worker to enforce his or her right to protection. Denied knowledge of the legal requirements, workers are very much at a disadvantage when dealing with management. Furthermore, as a result of the secrecy provisions in the Factories Act, workers have no right to hear the outcome of any investigation they may have requested. They do not even have the legal right to know if the investigation they requested has been instituted. The workers, therefore, who are intimately concerned with the maintenance of standards, are excluded from setting and monitoring those standards.

Mineworkers and mining diseases

South Africa has a poor record of mine safety compared with other countries. Over the years 1974-77 (*see Table XII*) at least two workers died every day, on average, in the mines. These figures exclude deaths as a result of occupational diseases or during 'riots'.

In 1982, only one person was employed in South Africa to ensure the occupational safety of 700,000 people working on the mines. The Medical Bureau for Occupational Diseases, whose 1980-81 report was tabled in April that year, reported that while in theory there should be three inspectors, there were at the time only two posts, one of which was vacant. Unattractive salary scales and the constant travelling entailed made it difficult to recruit staff. In consequence, regular inspections were not carried out and 'there are many places where the records of medical examinations and the quality of x-ray films fall short of the minimum standard required'.[22]

The accident rate in the gold mines has always tended to be particularly high, even in relation to the large numbers of workers involved. International exposure and criticism of conditions have made the multinational companies involved in the gold mining industry, in particular, sensitive on the issue, and steps have been taken to improve the image of South African mine safety.

In 1981 a spokesman for the Chamber of Mines claimed that South Africa was the most advanced country in the world in terms of the safety measures in its mines, and that on the international mines safety rating

TABLE XIII: Comparative figures for mine safety, 1973.

Country	Fatal Accidents per 1,000 Employees
Britain	0.43
U.S.A.	0.49
France	0.69
West Germany	0.69
Zambia	0.71
Kenya	0.80
South Africa – all mines	1.07
gold mines (whites)	1.05
gold mines (blacks)	1.57

Source: The depressed state of the African population under apartheid in the Republic of South Africa, by Diana Ellis & Julian R. Friedman, U.N. Centre Against Apartheid, Notes and Documents 24/76, December 1976.

scale, South Africa had nine five-star mines. Other member countries, including the US, Britain and Australia had no five-star mines. The spokesman nevertheless admitted that other South African gold mines were not scoring so highly, due to particularly difficult operating conditions, the extreme depth of the ore, and the 'relatively unsophisticated' work force.[23]

Mineworkers' diseases include tuberculosis (TB), silicosis, pneumoconiosis, chronic bronchitis and emphysema.

In 1978 it was reported that 570 out of 100,000 black miners had tuberculosis in the previous year.[24] In response the medical adviser to The Employment Bureau of Africa (TEBA, the recruiting arm of the Chamber of Mines, formerly WENELA) claimed that there was no connection between mining and TB and complained that the mines were the only industry obliged by law to contribute towards TB compensation for their workers.

Silicosis is the result of the inhalation of dust containing high concentrations of silica. Concentrations of up to 40 per cent have been measured in the gold mines. Silicosis is also common in coal mining. The disease becomes particularly serious when an infectious element such as TB is superimposed, leading to massive fibrosis of the lungs. The death rate from silicosis barely features in South African mining statistics because at the slightest suspicion of the disease the miner is immediately sent to hospital and subjected to a thorough medical examination. If the suspicion is confirmed and the miner is African, he will be dismissed and sent back to the reserves or other place of origin, where he will in all probability eventually die. The most that an African suffering from silicosis can expect in compensation is a small lump sum.[25]

46

In general, compensation for all diseases arising out of work in the mines varies according to population group. For Africans the established system does not differentiate between degrees of disablement or make any specific arrangements for payment to widows. For a compensatable disease other than TB an African miner qualifies for a lump sum payment of R1,000. If he has a compensatable disease plus TB, the compensation is R1,200. The compensation rates for TB alone are shown in Table XIV.

TABLE XIV: Compensation rates for tuberculosis contracted in the mines.

	Lump sum benefits (R)		
	White	Coloured	African
Tuberculosis	7,454	3,728	895
Certification in the first degree	17,889	8,945	1,491
Certification in the second degree	26,833	13,417	1,790

Note: These compensation rates are provided for under the Occupational Diseases in Mines and Works Act 1973. This Act applies solely to the mining industry and it removes a specific group of workers from the terms of the Workmen's Compensation Act 1941 as far as occupational diseases are concerned. It provides for lump sum benefits only and contains different provisions for three main population groups, defined in the Act as 'White', 'Coloured' and 'Black' ('African' in the Table).

The Workmen's Compensation Act 1941 covers all 'workmen' (male or female), irrespective of where they work or what they do. The definition of 'workmen' under the Act excludes persons whose earnings exceed R12,000 a year. Compensation rates under the Act are not affected by the population group of the worker concerned.

Source: Department of Mineral and Energy Affairs, *Report of the Commission of Inquiry into Compensation for Occupational Diseases in the Republic of South Africa*, 1981.

If an African miner dies while suffering from a compensatable disease other than TB, or a compensatable disease plus TB, the compensation received is only two thirds of what he would have received had he not died, or in the case of TB alone, only half. The amount to be paid is deposited at the Black Compensation Fund, from which the authority may at its *discretion* pay the amount to the dependants of the deceased.[26] This discretion means that widows may in fact never receive the compensation due to them.

Today, once an African has been certified as having a compensatable disease, he is immediately sent back to the bantustans or place of origin and is not allowed to work on a controlled mine again. In contrast, white miners who have contracted silicosis in the first degree may accept compensation until they are certified as having silicosis in the second degree, whereupon they are paid additional compensation, but have their certificates of fitness removed. Similarly a white tuberculotic may return to the mines provided he does no risk work.

Compensation in the mines is based on average monthly earnings (as it is in industry), but the scheme in force is different from and less comprehensive that that provided for under the Workmen's Compensation Act.[27]

The mines and the Medical Bureau for Occupational Diseases appear to pay little or no attention to black miners who leave the mines partially incapacitated. They receive no advice on alternative careers and there are no rehabilitation schemes; nor are less strenuous surface jobs found for them. Living conditions in the mine compounds involve large numbers of men sharing each room, often sleeping on concrete bunks. The overcrowded and insanitary conditions encourage TB and other infectious diseases.

In 1974, for example, there was an outbreak of cholera in Stilfontein and among miners employed in the Hartebeesfontein gold mine.[28] This was found to be due to contamination of drinking water in the acclimatisation centre. Mugs of water were left on the ground while the men performed strenuous exercises and sweated profusely. Contaminated droplets fell into the water. The situation was made worse by faecal contamination of the water reservoirs. The researchers also established that the great majority of new recruits became infected on the mines during their training period, having been tested and found negative for cholera prior to that.[29]

In May 1982, 400 workers at the Libanon gold mine in the West Rand contracted conjunctivitis, or 'pink eye'. The compound manager said that 50 new cases were being removed for treatment from the crowded hostels every day.[30]

Hospital and curative facilities for mineworkers who are injured or contract diseases are not the same for black as for white workers. In 1978 it was reported that a white workers' hospital in Parktown, Johannesburg, was to close because fewer white workers were being injured as more blacks were moving into the semi-skilled jobs.[31]

SOUTH AFRICA — MAIN TOWNS

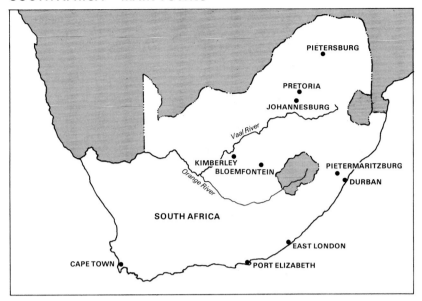

SOUTH AFRICA — THE BANTUSTANS

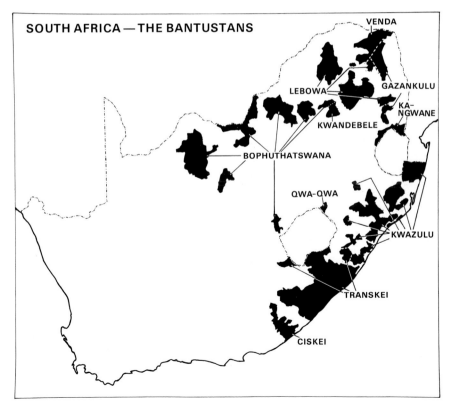

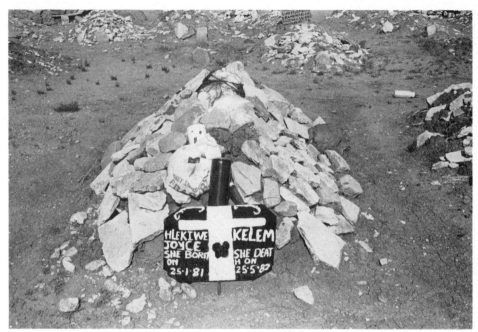

The grave of a 16-month-old baby at Ekuvukeni in the KwaZulu bantustan
Picture: Nancy Durrell-McKenna

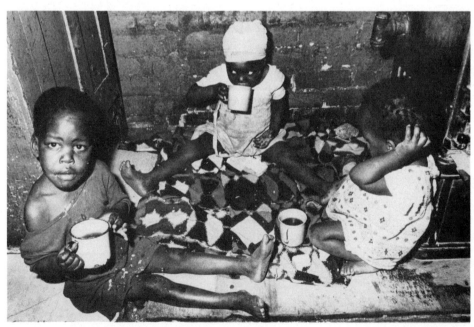

Many black children suffer from shortages of milk and other nutritious foods — these are drinking black tea
Picture: Nancy Durrell-McKenna

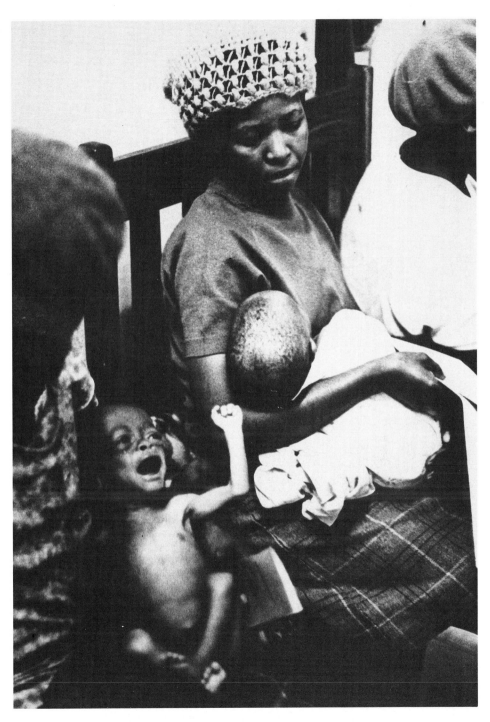

Malnourished infant in Baragwanath Hospital, Johannesburg   *Picture: Stan Winer*

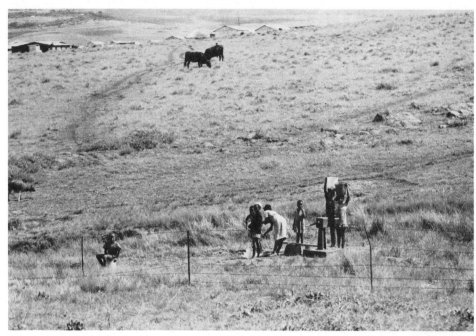

A water source in the Nondweni resettlement area, KwaZulu bantustan   Picture: Nancy Durrell-McKenna

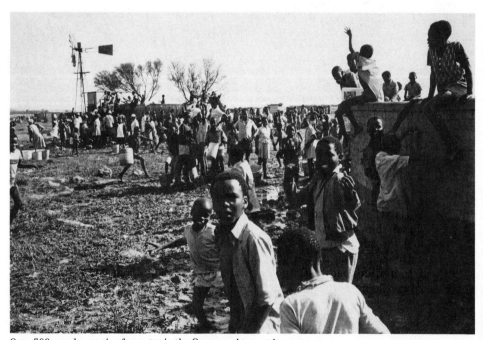

Over 500 people queuing for water in the Onverwacht resettlement area

Picture: Nancy Durrell-McKenna

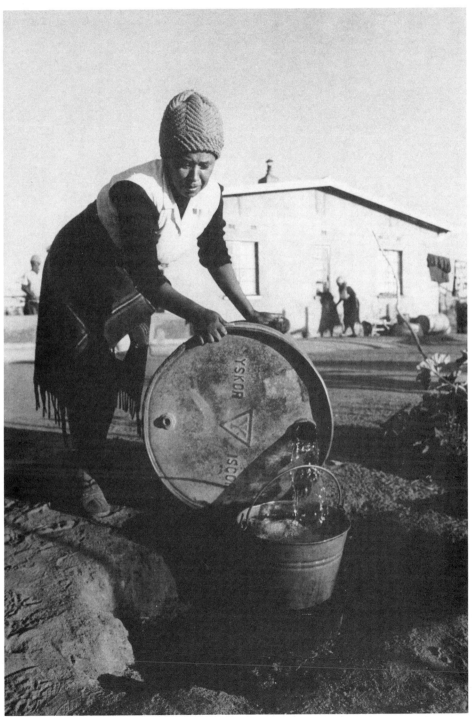

Water often has to be carried long distances and carefully conserved   Picture: Nancy Durrell-McKenna

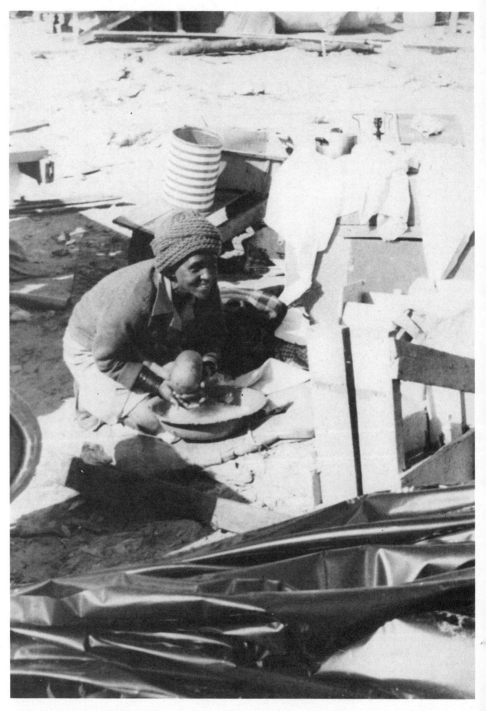

Making-do in a squatter camp　　　　　　　　　　　　　　　　*Picture: IDAF*

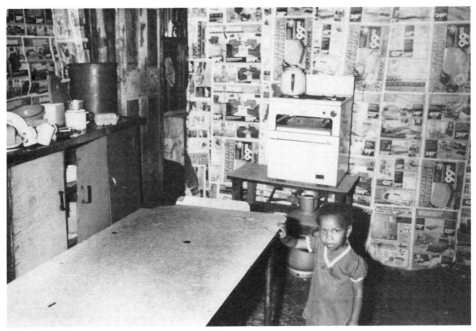

Inside a comparatively well-established squatter home in a Coloured area of the Cape
Picture: Nancy Durrell-McKenna

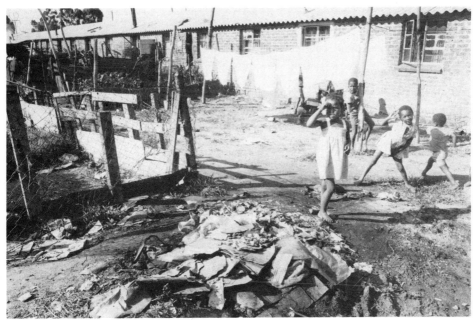

A hostel in Soweto, used by people who had lost other accommodation in flooding
Picture: Nancy Durrell-McKenna

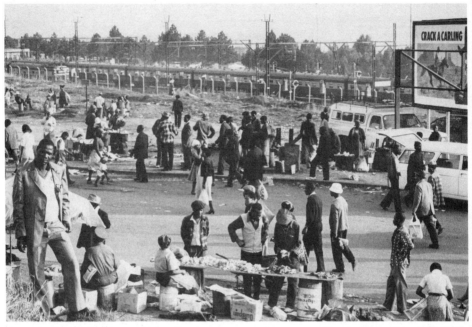

A street market in Soweto, outside a railway station   Picture: Nancy Durrell-McKenna

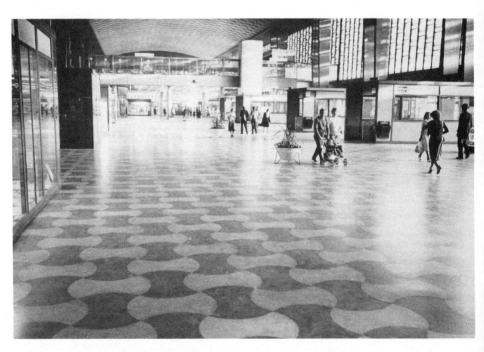

Inside a white railway station in Johannesburg   Picture: Nancy Durrell-McKenna

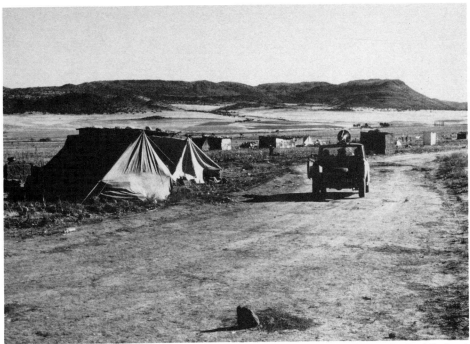

A resettlement camp　　　　　　　　　　　　　　*Picture: Roeland Kerbosch*

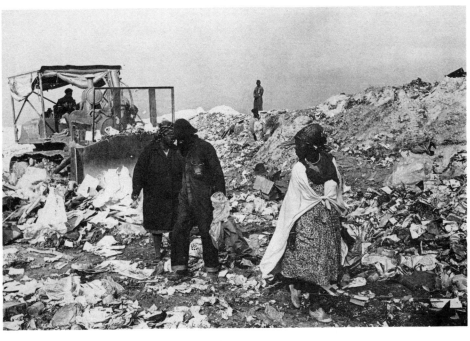

Scavenging on the rubbish tips of Johannesburg　　　　　*Picture: Rick Kollektiff*

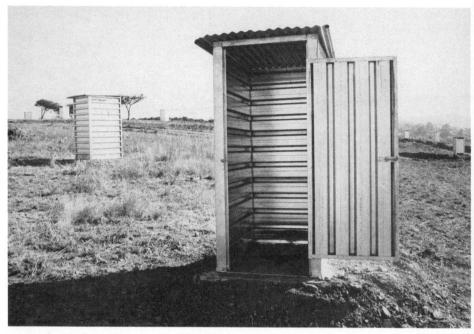

Latrines may be the only facility provided for those removed under the bantustan programme — a resettlement area in Inanda, Natal   *Picture: IDAF*

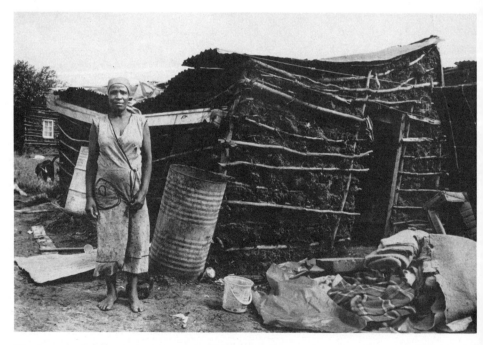

Housing in the Slangspruit squatter camp outside Maritzburg   *Picture: IDAF*

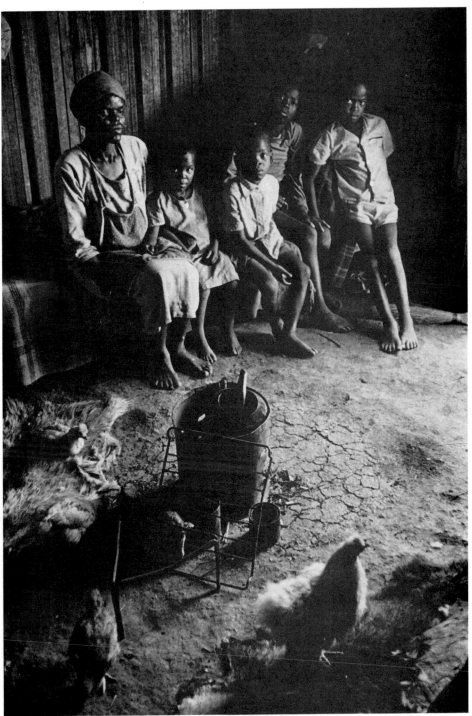

Inside a shelter provided by the state at a resettlement camp   *Picture: IDAF*

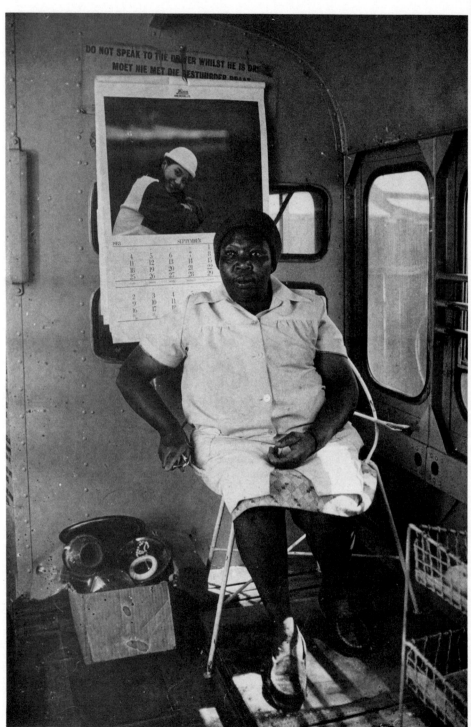

This woman moved into an abandoned bus after being removed from her home in Alexandra township

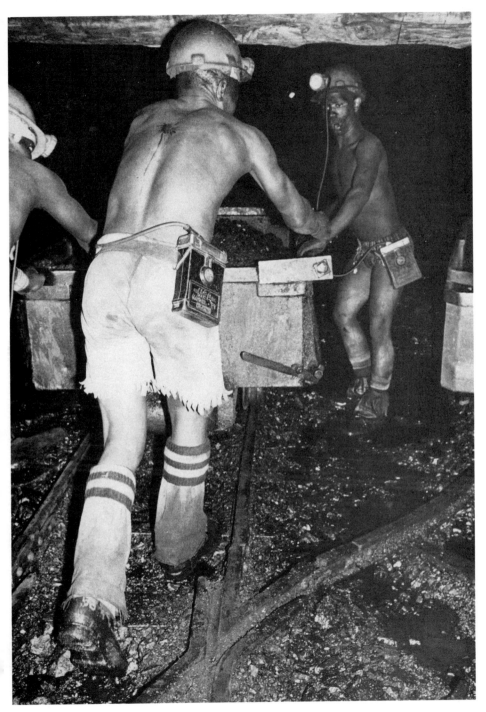

Working conditions in the mines   *Picture: Nancy Durrell-McKenna*

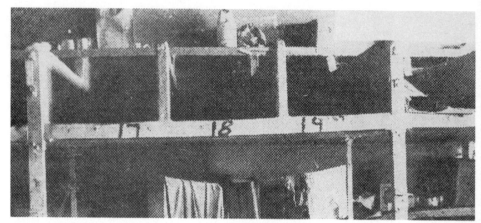

Concrete bunks provided for workers in a hostel compound. Some firms provide mattresses for their employees

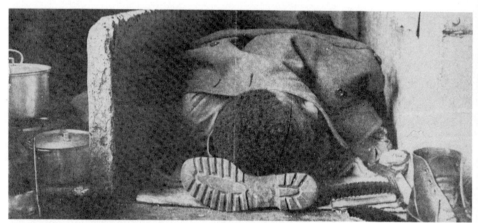

A migrant worker sleeps surrounded by possessions and cooking pots

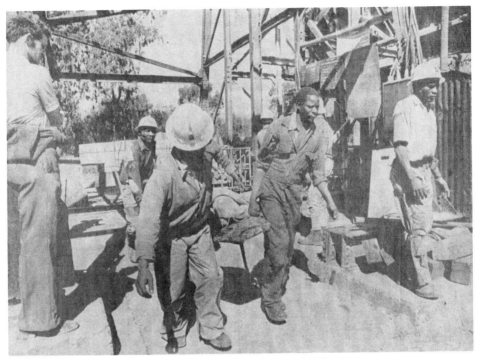

The bodies of those who died are brought to the surface after a mining disaster

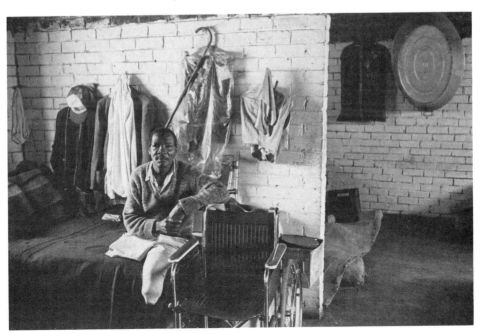

A disabled worker accommodated in a transit camp in Soweto   *Picture: Nancy Durrell-McKenna*

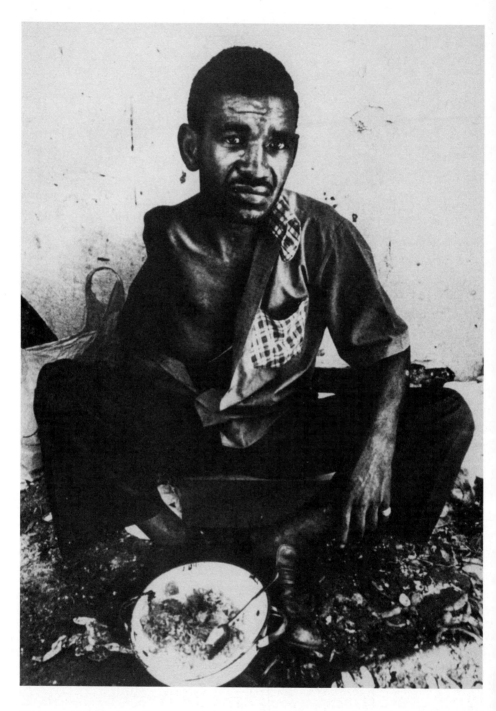

This manual labourer lost his arm in a road accident. He received no compensation, lost both his job and his rented lodging, and was forced to turn to begging and scavenging to survive Picture: Steve Bloom

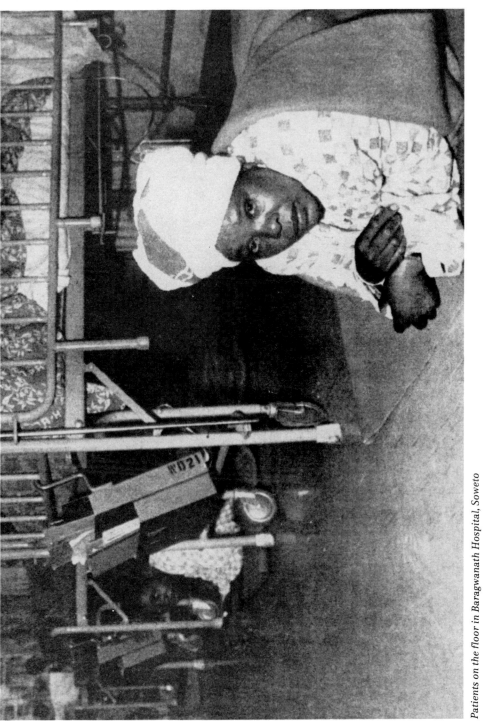

Patients on the floor in Baragwanath Hospital, Soweto

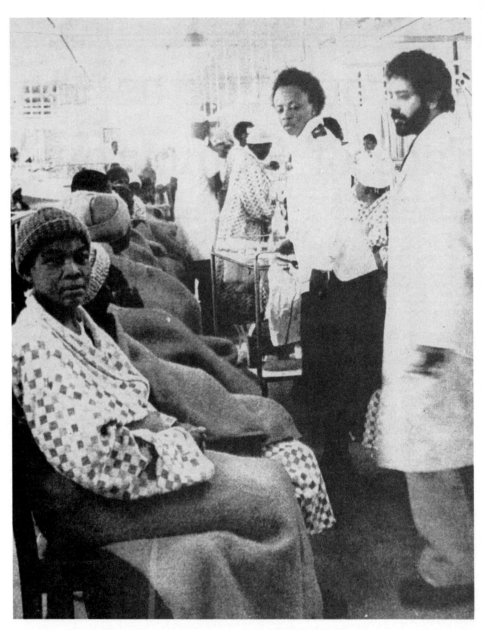

Doctors and nurses work in overcrowded conditions in Baragwanath

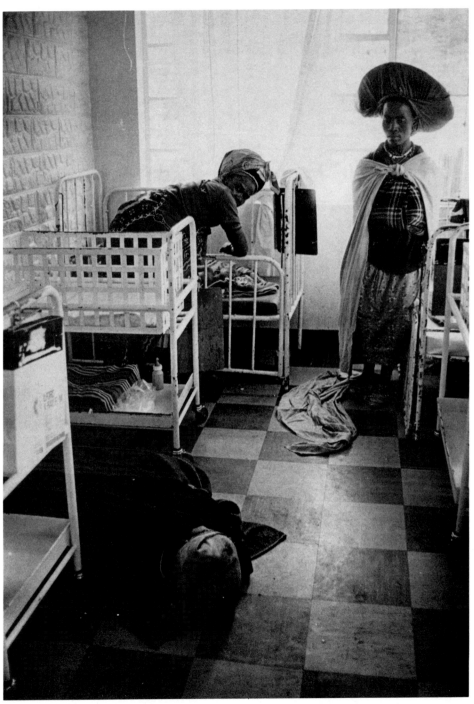

A ward in a Scottish mission hospital, Tugela River

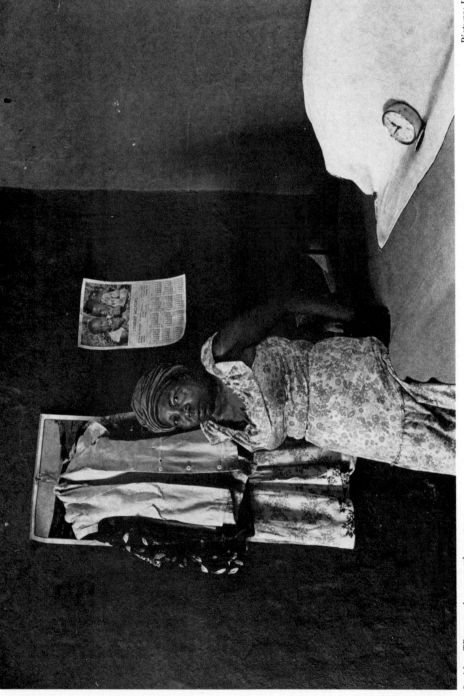

Inside a TB centre in a resettlement area

Four families live in a room constructed from makeshift materials in this TB centre in a resettlement area

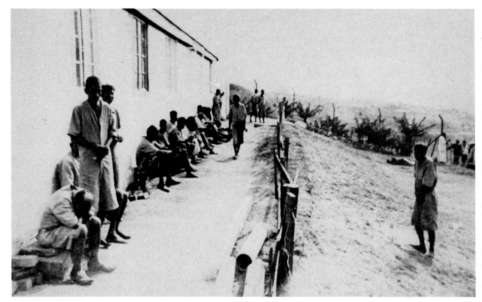

The compound of a mental hospital   *Picture: IDAF*

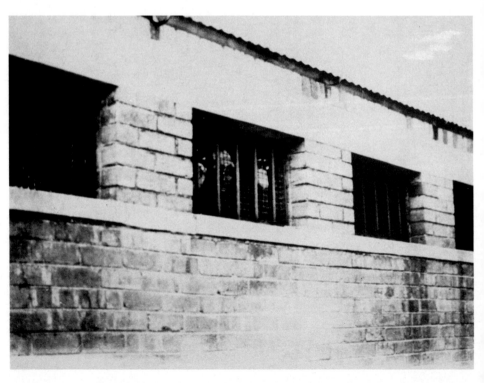

A patient looks out through the barred window of a mental hospital   *Picture: IDAF*

Picture: IDAF

Patients in a mental hospital

Picture: IDAF

A mental patient who died is carried away for burial by other hospital inmates.

6. Mental Health

Mental institutions — the Smith, Mitchell scandal

In 1974-75, the South African press exposed the existence of a chain of privately owned institutions accommodating thousands of black mental patients. The majority of these patients were detained involuntarily through a perfunctory medical and legal procedure. The institutions were described as 'human warehouses' by the President of the South African National Council for Mental Health, and as the South African version of Dickensian workhouses by a journalist who in 1978 accidentally gained access to one of them.[1]

Details of the way in which these mental institutions were controlled and managed began to emerge in the furore which followed their discovery. Private enterprise, in the shape of Smith, Mitchell and Company Ltd., of Johannesburg, was found to be running the institutions as a profit-making venture, in collaboration with the South African Department of Health. Smith, Mitchell and Co. was registered as an accounting firm and functioned as an agent for 89 different companies, 12 of which were psychiatric institutions. One of the companies, Protea Ltd., specialised in hospital supplies and had been directly implicated in the management of Smith, Mitchell institutions. The biggest shareholder in Protea was found to be the Standard Bank of South Africa, in turn controlled by Chase Manhattan Bank of New York.[2]

Protea was chaired until 1976 by David Tabatznik. He was responsible for the establishment of the Smith, Mitchell institutions by leasing old mining compounds formerly used for tuberculosis patients. Under a contractual agreement with the State, these institutions accommodated psychiatric patients when the state institutions became full or for long term custodial care, the State paying Smith, Mitchell and Co. a fee per patient per day.

In 1979 it was also disclosed that Connie Mulder, the former South African cabinet minister who resigned in the wake of the South African Information Department scandal, had financial interests in several mental homes. In the early 1960s Mulder was, with Tabatznik, one of the directors of the Randfontein Non-White Sanatorium and the Rand West Sanatorium in Transvaal. Dr. Mulder resigned his directorship on becoming a cabinet minister in 1968, but retained shares in seven other Smith, Mitchell companies.[3]

Little information has been available on psychiatric patients in private institutions except through questions in parliament. As far as mental patients in state institutions are concerned, the Secretary of Health (and up to 1970 the Commissioner of Health) is compelled by law to provide an annual report.

Official figures given in parliament for the years 1976 and 1977 (*see Table XV*) showed that the majority of patients in private mental hospitals were African, while in the state institutions, the majority were white. A comparatively small number of white patients (less than 10 per cent of the total) were being treated in private institutions, while Africans were roughly equally divided between these and the state hospitals. According to the Department of Health the State was directly responsible for 20 psychiatric hospitals and licensed 37 other institutions run by private companies, medical practitioners and charitable organisations.[4]

TABLE XV: Psychiatric patients in mental institutions, 1977 and 1980.

Population group	State institutions 1977	1980	Other (private) 1977	1980	Total 1977	1980
White	7,830	7,064	707	609	8,537	7,673
Coloured	2,763	2,462	483	449	3,246	2,911
Indian	150	156	260	372	410	528
African	5,467	4,707	5,632	5,034	11,099	9,741
Total	16,210	14,389	7,082	6,464	23,292	20,853

Note: The figures are as at the ends of the years in question.

Sources: Debates, 8.3.78; *SAIRR,* 1981, p.402.

In 1980-81 the official picture as far as the numbers of beds in private hospitals were concerned remained roughly the same: there were 656 beds for white psychiatric patients, 500 for Coloured, 250 for Indian and 5,845 for African patients.[5]

In fact, the real figure for the number of mental patients in the private, Smith, Mitchell and Co. institutions is much higher than this — probably because several of them are situated in the bantustans and so do not feature in the official statistics. The Smith, Mitchell institutions accommodate over 10,000 Africans and several hundred white, Coloured and Indian patients (*see Table XVI*). One report in 1980 suggested that they might hold over 20,000 patients.[6] The South African government has granted Smith, Mitchell and Co. sole rights to mental institutions in the bantustans.[7]

The South African government subsidises white mental patients at a higher rate than black patients. In 1977, the Minister disclosed that the daily subsidy varied from R1.22 to R4.31 per patient, 'depending upon the level of service rendered'.[8]

The shocking consequences of racial discrimination in psychiatric hospital care were uncovered by, *inter alia,* the American Psychiatric Association (APA). In September 1978 the APA sent a delegation to South Africa to investigate conditions in private mental institutions, at the invitation of the South African Department of Health and Smith, Mitchell and Co. themselves.[9] International opinion had been alerted to the scandal by this time, through the publication the year before of a report by the World Health Organisation.[10]

The APA reported that the latest subsidy figures for mental patients ranged from R1.70 per day for black to R7 a day for whites. The delegation found that between 15 and 20 Africans were being sent to the Smith, Mitchell institutions every day. Many black patients were first sent to state institutions for 'observation' and then referred to the Smith, Mitchell institutions. This was often done without adequate screening processes but simply to relieve the overcrowded conditions in the state hospitals. The figures given for 'discharges' from the state institutions may be inflated by these kind of referrals. The APA found that relatives were frequently not even contacted prior to patients being transferred in this way.[11]

Initial admission to mental hospitals is insufficiently regulated in the view of experts, particularly with regard to Africans. They may be admitted in a manner which would be deemed intolerable if applied to whites: Professor J. H. Robbertze, head of the Clinical Psychology Department at the University of Pretoria (and incidentally the President of the South African National Council for Mental Health) pointed out that patients might be kept for 'indefinite periods' in the Smith, Mitchell institutions.[12]

The conditions in these institutions were described as appalling. They were situated in old mining compounds with high wire fences and wire mesh windows. The patients lived in primitive conditions, sleeping on grass mats on a cement floor — in some cases the mats had been made by the patients themselves. There was an almost complete lack of basic facilities such as toilet paper and bed linen, according to the American Psychiatric Association. There was discrimination in the clothing and food provided for black and white patients. At one institution the Association found that black patients had rioted over the poor quality food provided while white patients were more satisfied with their food than 'most hospital patients in the United States.'[13]

Even more disturbing was the fact that the majority of black patients in the Smith, Mitchell institutions told the visiting American psychiatrists that they had been beaten and assaulted by the staff or had witnessed assaults on other patients by the staff. The Association concluded 'that violence grows out of the mentality of Apartheid which treats non-whites as inferiors and accepts the degrading of their humanity as a matter of course'.[14]

The delegation found that the 10,000 black patients in the institutions they visited were not receiving adequate medical and psychiatric attention. One sign of this was a four-fold excess of deaths from tuberculosis amongst African mental patients. The Association reported that the 'most shocking finding' of their entire investigation was the high number of needless deaths amongst the patients due to lack of medical care. Most of the patients interviewed had never had a physical examination during their stay in the institutions.

Furthermore, the results of brief mental status examinations conducted by the team were often totally incompatible with the recorded diagnosis, thus confirming their view that the majority of patients had been admitted without adequate screening procedures.

The Smith, Mitchell institutions claimed that they gave the patients 'occupational therapy'. This term seemed rather misleading in the light of the fact that in the institution, the Springfield Sanatorium catering for Indian patients, inmates were made to work 11 hours a day. Patients were paid the equivalent of R2-10 a month, mainly in the form of cigarettes or sweets. It was claimed that the profits from this labour were used for improving services, but this was not confirmed by the APA delegates, who stated that 'little, if any of the revenue gathered from the sale of goods seems to be returned to the patients.'[15]

Smith, Mitchell and Co. would appear to make substantial profits by using patients' labour for building, maintenance and repairs of the institutions themselves, and by sub-contracting patients to other firms. While state mental patients in other countries also work, the fact that Smith, Mitchell is a private company means that any work done by the patients tends either to reduce its costs or boost institutional income, thus increasing overall profits.

Overall, the APA delegation's investigation convinced the Association that
there is good reason for international concern about black psychiatric patients in South Africa. We found unacceptable medical practices that resulted in needless deaths of black South Africans. Medical and psychiatric care for blacks was grossly inferior to that for whites. We

found that apartheid has a destructive impact on families, social institutions and the mental health of black South Africans. We believe that these findings substantiate allegations of social and political abuse of psychiatry in South Africa.[16]

TABLE XVI: Psychiatric institutions run by Smith, Mitchell and Co.

Institution	White	Indian	Inmates Coloured	African	n/k
1. Allanridge*				400	
2. East Rand			500		
3. Ekhlengeni*				1,200	
4. Majestic Hotel	170				
5. Poloko*				1,200	
6. Randfontein (male)				3,600	
7. Randfontein (female)				1,490	
8. Simmer					295
9. Springfield		250			
10. Struisbult	100				
11. Thabamoopo*				1,200	
12. Turrets	125				
13. Waverly				755	
14. Witpoort	380				
Total	775	250	500	9,845	295

n/k – not known.

Notes: Institutions noted *, accommodating a total of 4,000 African patients, are located in bantustans.

No new institutions are known to have been established since May 1975.

Source: Statement by Minister of Health, in reply to a parliamentary question, *Debates*, 2.5.75.

The state response

The initial exposure inside South Africa of the Smith, Mitchell institutions provoked a public outcry. In 1976 the government temporarily withheld its subsidy from the company and after the issue had been discussed in parliament Tabatznik resigned as a director. The government's next reaction was to introduce the Mental Health Amendment Act of 1976. This was far from being a reform.

Under the headline 'Law to protect mental patients' an article in the South African press explained that the government was 'taking steps to protect mental patients against the intrusions into their privacy by magazines and other publications'.[17] The object of the Act was to prevent conditions in mental institutions from being publicly discussed and criticised. The Act dealt specifically with the dissemination of information about mental institutions in South Africa and prohibited the taking of photographs or sketches of institutions and patients by anyone who was not a member of the Newspaper Press Union of South Africa or who had not been authorised by the Secretary of State. The Department of Health claimed that the 'smear campaign' had spread to the 'foreign press'.

The Mental Health Amendment Act also prohibited the publication 'in any manner whatsoever' of 'false information concerning detention, treatment, behaviour or experience in an institution of any patient . . . or concerning the administration of any institution.' Persons who contravened the Act would be guilty of an offence and liable on conviction to a fine of R1,000 or imprisonment without the option of a fine, or both.

Thus while incriminating individuals deemed to be divulging 'false information' and who had not taken 'reasonable' steps to verify such information, the same law prohibited such offenders from access to methods of verifying information.

After all the furore it was reported in 1977 that R60 million was to be spent on five psychiatric hospitals including a hospital for Coloured patients at Mitchells Plain in Cape Town, and four hospitals for African patients at Mamelodi, Vereeniging, Daveyton, and Soweto, providing a total of 5,000 beds, to replace the existing Smith, Mitchell institutions.[18] The latter continued to function, however, the reports of the ill-treatment and poor conditions of patients persisted, and international concern grew. (By the beginning of 1984, moreover, it appeared that the five new psychiatric hospitals had still not been built.)

State mental hospitals

The American Psychiatric Association reported that examination of the records in the state mental hospitals they visited suggested that many black patients did not receive adequate medical and psychiatric evaluation or care before transfer to the Smith, Mitchell institutions. This was despite the fact that the Mental Health Act required a report on each patient's current medical status. The Association also had reason to believe that 'acutely ill' black patients were being transferred from state hospitals to the Smith, Mitchell institutions. They found an enormous discrepancy between facilities for black and white patients in the state hospitals, describing those provided for whites as 'comparing favourably with the best American hospitals'.[19]

Overall, there are gross disparities in the numbers of beds available in psychiatric hospitals for the members of different population groups. The World Health Organisation reported that the total number of psychiatric beds worked out at 2.55 per 1,000 whites (or one bed for each 392 people) and 0.76 beds per 1,000 blacks (Coloured, Indian, and African) (i.e. one bed for each 1,316 people).[20]

54

For mentally retarded people, one newspaper gave the following bed:population ratios for the year 1976: African — 1:4,296; Indian — 1:3,286; Coloured — 1:989; White — 1:488.[21]

During 1980, the Minister of Health stated that it was his department's policy to phase out mental institutions run by private organisations. To achieve this, additional funds had been approved for the current financial year to expedite the provision of 540 beds in the Eastern Cape area. Over the 1979-84 period the Department of Public Works planned to tender for five institutions in Soweto, Pretoria, Queenstown, Bloemfontein and Port Elizabeth (either new or additions to existing buildings), to provide a total of 2,570 new beds. In future, mental institutions would include a separate complex for the mentally retarded.[22]

It would appear that these plans proceeded slowly, however. In 1982 it was reported that a 932-bed psychiatric hospital for Africans was planned for Port Elizabeth, but work would only start in 1988 for estimated completion in 1992. The estimated tender date for the hospitals in Bloemfontein and Soweto was 1984. No final decision had been taken about the accommodation of mentally ill Coloured people in this area.[23]

While little detailed information is available, facilities and treatment for black psychiatric patients who do manage to gain admission to state hospitals would seem to leave much to be desired. In 1982 it was reported that at least 10 mentally disturbed patients were admitted to Baragwanath Hospital in Soweto every day, but that the psychiatric service at the hospital consisted of only two psychiatrists, each of whom consulted on one day a week.[24]

The situation seemed little changed in 1983, when a press report stated that a clinical psychologist attended to patients for the entire hospital, four times a week. Journalists who visited Baragwanath found that there were no special facilities for psychiatric cases and these were simply 'farmed out' to various wards, ending up with about five psychiatric patients in each ward, mixed together with those with other complaints. Doctors administered drugs to the psychiatric patients, and if their condition deteriorated, they would be referred to Sterkfontein Hospital. Before that happened however, it might be found necessary to tie psychiatric patients to their beds to prevent them from thrashing about. 'Sometimes they become wild and chase the nurses,' one sister said. 'It is very hard for us. And we must also always wear a smile for the patients.' Because there were too few beds, psychiatric patients, dazed by drugs, often wandered off and got lost in the hospital grounds. Nursing staff pinned notes to their hospital gowns, to tell those who found them which wards they should be returned to.[25]

Psychiatric personnel

The 1981 annual report of the Department of Health admitted that institutional services for psychiatric patients suffered from a shortage of personnel. The report gave a figure of 4,596 for the total number of specialists and staff associated with psychiatric services (*see Tables XVII and XVIII*). Others work in private practice. During 1982 there were only eight black psychiatrists in South Africa — seven Indian and one Coloured. The first African psychiatrist was currently being trained at the Medical University of South Africa (Medunsa) in Bophuthatswana, and a second African doctor would begin psychiatric training at the Hillbrow hospital in 1983.[26]

The lack of black medical personnel means that those dealing with psychiatric patients often cannot speak their language, nor understand their cultural background. The American Psychiatric Association delegation reported that none of the psychiatrists in the institutions they visited could speak an African language.

Out-patient care

Up until 1960 practically no out-patient services or community health care were available for the mentally ill in South Africa. By 1975, the South African National Council for Mental Health operated a total of 24 out-patient clinics with 40,000 attendances annually, but no breakdown of this figure for the different population groups was available. There were 220,743 attendances at state clinics in the same year.[27] The total number of registered out-patients in 1975 was given as 56,282 at state clinics and 18,000 at Mental Health Society clinics.[28] The authorities claim that since the advent of psychotropic drugs the policy has been to limit hospitalisation and shift emphasis to community care. This may or may not indicate an improvement in care for the mentally ill for, in the absence of adequate facilities, it may well be a way of simply reducing state expenditure.

Types of mental illness

A sharp increase in the number of Africans certified and detained in mental institutions was perceived in the 1960s, a period in which the bantustan policy was being accelerated and thousands of people were being forcibly removed. The uprooting of people and the disruption of family life made it difficult for the mentally ill to be cared for at home by relatives.

In 1980, around 5,000 mentally retarded people were being cared for by their families, according to the head of the Genetic Services Division of the Department of Health and Welfare. Out of a total of around 23,000 patients in mental hospitals, 7,000 were diagnosed as mental retardates. Of these, 4,500 were in state institutions and the remainder in subsidised private institutions.[29]

TABLE XVII: Personnel associated with psychiatric services, 1980-81.

	1981	*1980*
Medical personnel		
Psychiatrist	72	47
General practitioner/		
registrar	55	72
Nursing personnel		
Registered and enrolled	1,608	1,874
Assistants	2,713	2,698
Social workers	26	33
Paramedical personnel		
Clinical psychologist	42	41
Occupational therapist	47	39
Physiotherapist	7	8
Pharmacist	26	21
Total	4,596	4,833

Source: Department of Health annual report for 1981, cited in *SAIRR*, 1982, p.538.

TABLE XVIII: Available mental health personnel in South Africa, 1964-76.

Year	Population	Psychiatrists	Clinical psychologists	Psychiatric nurses	Social workers in mental health
1964	19.5 mil	82	40	674	37
1970	22.4 mil	134	92	896	50
1975	25.5 mil	164	191	2,079	97
1976	26.1 mil	167	238	2,779	99

Source: Professor J. H. Robbertze, *Mental health priorities in South Africa,* paper presented to SALDRU/SAMST Conference on the economics of health care in Southern Africa, University of Cape Town, September 1978, in *Hunger, Work and Health,* ed. Francis Wilson and Gill Westcott, Ravan Press, Johannesburg, 1980.

Facilities for the mentally retarded are, as in other branches of the health services, different for white and black. There is a great shortage of residential care for mentally retarded African patients and special training and education services for them are practically non-existent. Caring for them at home means an additional burden for black families already coping with the problems of the pass laws, low wages and poor and over-crowded living conditions.

A total of 750 mentally retarded children were found to be accommodated in the Smith, Mitchell institutions. In 1975, four special classes for retarded African children were opened in primary schools.[30]

The officially recorded incidence of other types of mental illness and their treatment — personality disorders, psychoses and psychoneuroses, dementia etc. — varies between the population groups. Figures for the types of mental illness in patients discharged from state institutions in 1975, as given by the Chief Psychiatrist, revealed that neuroses constituted 21 per cent of first admissions for whites and only two per cent of admissions for other groups. This does not mean to say that neuroses are uncommon in other population groups, but rather that the limited facilities available mean that only the most serious and urgent cases can be dealt with in the institutions. Amongst blacks, according to some sources, schizophrenia accounts for almost two thirds of all first admissions while toxic and exhaustion psychosis (i.e. secondary to infections, alcoholism, vitamin deficiency etc.) account for one sixth and so-called epileptic psychosis for one twelfth.[31] However, a survey of 104 psychiatric patients at the Mpilo Hospital, Bulawayo, Zimbabwe (then Rhodesia) in 1976 revealed that 22.1 per cent of patients were schizophrenic, 20.2 per cent were suffering from toxic psychosis and 20.2 per cent from depression. Only 4.8 per cent were epileptics. Some of the organic conditions presenting with toxic and exhaustion psychosis are pneumonia, typhoid fever, pulmonary tuberculosis, pellagra psychosis and confusional states due to alcohol or dagga (marijuana).[32]

It has been estimated that over 50 per cent of black mental patients admitted to a Pretoria hospital in 1969 were suffering from dementia due to pellagra, a vitamin deficiency disease.[33] This condition presents 26,000 cases annually according to a survey carried out in the late 1960s by the National Nutrition Institute.[34] A survey reported in 1980 of the Hewu district of the Ciskei bantustan showed that 33 per cent of the adult population had pellagra.[35] With vitamin treatment the condition may be reversed.

The treatment which those with mental disorders receive in South Africa, particularly black patients, may well be inappropriate to their needs. The American Psychiatric Association gained the impression that many of the patients admitted with so-called toxic psychosis were actually suffering from functional psychosis (a psychiatric rather than a physical condition). This could have been diagnosed by more careful evaluation. The APA claimed that the more sophisticated South African psychiatrists agreed with them. The APA also questioned the need for involuntary and long-term confinement for epileptics with no mental retardation or other complicating neurological or psychiatric conditions.[36] Most South African psychiatric personnel apparently share a popular belief that violence and epilepsy are correlated. While this is often used as a reason to incarcerate epileptics, it is not borne out by research. In this regard it is interesting to note that only 4.8 per cent of psychiatric patients at the Mpilo Hospital (see above) were classified as epileptics.

In December 1980 the Society for Safety in Mental Healing expressed similar fears, when they questioned the need to confine epileptics, the mentally retarded, alcoholics and drug addicts in mental institutions. They also said that urgent amendments were needed to laws governing the treatment of mental patients, to prevent those awaiting transfer to mental institutions, and others who were not criminals, from being confined in police cells.[37]

The poverty-stricken environment characteristic of the majority of South Africa's black population encourages the incidence of mental illnesses which have organic causes. Besides the vitamin deficiency disease pellagra, protein-calorie malnutrition in children starves the growing brain of essential nutrients and can lead to mental retardation. Infections such as tuberculosis are important causes of mental illness, not only because of actual brain damage due to cerebral infection, but also as a result of toxic and exhaustion psychosis.[38]

The laws and practices of the apartheid system itself are sources of fear, stress, anxiety and trauma for millions of black South Africans. The migrant labour system and the pass laws destroy family life and create insecurity and worry about the welfare of children, parents, partners and other relatives. Lack of education and training opportunities for black people, combined with job reservation practices, create frustration and resentment. Above all, apartheid society is inherently violent, relying as it does on the use of force to retain power and privilege in the hands of a minority. Such an environment must tend to undermine mental health.

Suicide

The stressful situation in which South Africans find themselves is reflected in the figures for suicide.

In 1982, Sam Bloomberg, the founder-chairman of the South African Suicide Prevention Centre and Suicides Anonymous, warned that suicide was the fastest-growing cause of death in South Africa. Although no reliable statistics for attempted suicide were available, he estimated that 150,000 people considered taking their own lives every year. Nearly 3,000 succeeded in doing so.[39]

Bloomberg said that suicide was now the third most common cause of death among white South Africans under the age of 20. Among black people, where in the past suicide had been almost unknown, the suicide rate was fast approaching that of whites. He predicted that these trends would continue, exacerbated by mass unemployment, insecurity and political pressures.[40]

In 1948, when the Nationalist government came to power and the constitutional doctrine of apartheid was officially launched, there was a sharp increase in the suicide rate (see Table XIX). It is thought that this was most probably due to the anticipated reclassification of population groups. The race classification and mixed marriage laws were among the first apartheid statutes to be introduced by the Nationalist party.

TABLE XIX: Suicide rates, 1947-48.

Population group	Suicide rate per 100,000 population	
	1947	1948
African	8.8	18.1
Coloured	15.8	36.3
Indian	20.5	23.6
White	17.5	19.2

Source: Fatima Meer, Race and Suicide in South Africa, 1976.

Suicide rates remained high. In 1976, the white suicide rate in Johannesburg was described by Professor G. K. Engelbrecht of the Rand Afrikaans University as the second highest in the world, following West Berlin.[41] A total of 4,000 people were reported to have killed themselves in the city in 1976 (the year of the Soweto uprisings), while 100,000 had attempted to do so.[42] The South African representative of the International Association for Suicide Prevention was quoted as saying that whites were affected by two main problems — aggression and despair. Fear played an important role. Suicidals talked 'confusedly of the blacks coming down from the north to take over the country and say they want to die before that happens'.[43]

'Suicide and self-inflicted injury' was listed by medical researchers as the tenth most important cause of death among white South Africans for the year 1976, with an overall rate of 15.1 deaths per 100,000. (Ischaemic heart diseases, the most important cause, accounted for 217.4 deaths per 100,000). The suicide rate was much higher among white men (23.4 per 100,000) than among white women (6.9 per 100,000). Suicide did not feature among the ten most important causes of death for the remaining three main population groups.[44]

Alcoholism

The annual *per capita* consumption of alcohol among whites in South Africa is one of the highest in the western world. Three-quarters of all white South Africans drink alcohol, consuming 82 million litres in 1975. In 1977, total spending on liquor in South Africa amounted to R1,382 million, R32 more than the defence budget for that year. There were estimated to be 100,000 alcoholics and the rate of consumption was rising.[45]

In a report to a health conference in September 1978 on alcoholism in the Western Cape, it was estimated that the incidence of addictive alcoholism among Coloured people in the Western Cape was of the order of six to eight per cent and that in total (white and Coloured males) at least 22 per cent of the men living in Cape Town and its environs drank excessively.[46] It is not surprising that alcoholism amongst Cape Coloured people is so high considering living conditions and, particularly, the treatment of farm workers in the Cape who are paid with wine as part of their wages. Under the so-called 'dop' (tot) system, farm workers are given a tin filled with locally brewed wine, some farmers giving 10 'dops' daily plus two bottles to take home. Workers thus become addicted and dependent on their employers.[47]

Amongst whites excessive drinking is reflected in the number of traffic and pedestrian accidents in which alcohol plays a role.

There are no reliable figures for the incidence of alcoholism amongst urban Africans, but some indicators of increasing alcohol consumption are the steady increase in liver cirrhosis amongst blacks and the increase in the annual *per capita* consumption of so-called 'Bantu beer'. Drinking of methylated spirits by alcoholics is increasing because of its cheapness and availability.[48]

Some of the factors contributing to excessive drinking are poverty, job reservation, poor living conditions, lack of recreational facilities, and the group areas regulations. Alcoholism amongst better educated black people is the result of frustration as many cannot progress professionally owing to the laws and customs of apartheid. Amongst the migrant workers in the bleak hostels in the urban townships, liquor is a means of obliterating or at least softening the harsh reality of everyday life in which there is no home or family to return to after the day's work. In 1978 the West Rand Administration Board (WRAB) noted that the municipal beer halls were attacked by students in Soweto in 1976 in protest against liquor sales. A WRAB official was quoted as saying 'we build as the need arises.'[49] Soweto is largely run on the liquor profits made by WRAB.

In 1978 it was reported that 14.5 per cent of personal expenditure by urban Africans went on alcohol.[50] The scale of the problem was also noted by a visiting Assistant Professor at the School of Social Work at

61

Arizona State University who was quoted as saying that alcoholism amongst blacks in South Africa was more critical than in any other place he had visited.[51] In 1982, a Durban welfare worker claimed that up to 75 per cent of marriages broke up in the townships as a direct result of alcoholism. Marshall Ngidi, who was also information officer for the South African National Council on Alcoholism (SANCA), said that for many black men, it had become a way of life to spend the whole weekend drinking. Many husbands stopped handing over any money at all to their wives because of their drinking problem.[52]

To summarise, the apartheid system, involving the forced removal of over three million people, the splitting of families and the pervasive climate of police harassment, is hardly the climate for the development of psychiatric and mental health. The psychiatric facilities provided for the black population are inadequate and poor in quality. Patients have been laid open to abuse in private institutions which, far from providing therapy and support, have been used as cheap labour camps. The question which must arise is why it was found necessary to pass the Mental Health Amendment Act of 1976 if there was nothing to hide.

In their report on mental health care in South Africa the World Health Organisation concluded '. . . such policies are however part and parcel of the overall doctrine of apartheid and radical improvements in the present situation in the mental health services are inconceivable as long as apartheid remains in force.'[53]

7. Health Services

The present structure of the health service in South Africa dates back to the passing of the Public Health Act in 1919. The central government controls a minority of hospital services including a number of tuberculosis institutions and mental hospitals, but most of the curative services, particularly the hospitals, fall under the control of the different provincial administrations. Public health measures fall under the central government with the exception of environmental controls, social health services and control of communicable diseases. These are delegated to the local authorities in the provinces.

The net result is that there is very little correlation between preventative and curative services.

In recent years, some of the health services in the bantustan areas (most of which had been provided by mission stations and churches) have been placed under the authority of the local 'governments'. Up to 1970 all the health services fell under the control of the South African Department of Health. Since that year the bantustan health services, other than those in the 'independent' bantustans, have been under the jurisdiction of the Department of Bantu Administration and Development (now Co-operation and Development), with the South African Department of Health acting on their behalf. These changes in the statutory responsibilities have not altered the overall structure.

In the early 1940s discussions took place regarding the establishment of a National Health Service, but with the change in government in 1948 and the coming into power of the Nationalists, the idea was abandoned and funds for the health service were drastically cut.[1] The health service today is a mixture of statutory, private, and charitable facilities. The curative health service takes three main forms. In the large cities and towns the general practitioner is often the first form of contact. The patient pays a fee, or if covered by a medical aid scheme, is partially assisted with payment. Patients requiring further, more specialised care are then either referred to a hospital or private specialist, depending on income or preference. In other cases, particularly for those without access to a general practitioner or the money for the fee, the hospital casualty and/or out-patients department is the first contact. This is the usual route for black people and in cases of emergency.

Hospitals

Hospital attendance for blacks is a test of endurance requiring endless patience and fortitude — and this when the person could be very ill.

Patients are known to spend an entire day plus evening waiting for treatment at some busy major hospitals. A day at the hospital often means the loss of a day's pay as well. Some clinics have been set up in the townships to provide a quicker service, but these are badly staffed, often only with nurses, with a doctor coming in only a few hours a day. Patients who are seriously ill still have to go to the major hospitals.

In the rural areas, which are the worst off, the population is often served only by the mission hospitals to which many patients have to travel great distances. Few district surgeons are available. Some private practitioners are to be had, but these cater mainly for the white population.

In general white patients have better access to better facilities — less crowded hospitals, speedier referral, better equipped surgeries and so on. With few exceptions, all facilities are segregated, those for whites being amongst the best in the world and those for blacks being greatly inferior.

Some visiting doctors from abroad appear to be unaware of these discrepancies and praise conditions that their own patients and staff at home would find intolerable. Facilities at Baragwanath Hospital in Soweto, for example, have often been cited as an example of the superior medical care enjoyed by South African blacks compared to their counterparts elsewhere in Africa. The propaganda publications produced by the South African government give a glowing impression of conditions there, which is often mirrored in reports published abroad.

Baragwanath Hospital is in fact acutely overcrowded. Situated on the edge of Soweto, it has an estimated 2,500 beds which, together with eight clinics, serve the whole of Soweto, estimated population more than one million. In its 1981-82 financial year, Baragwanath treated 112,000 in-patients and 1,620,000 out-patients. In winter, bed occupancy in the medical and surgical wards can be up to 300 per cent and 250 per cent respectively. When a deputation from the Transvaal Provincial Council and the press visited the hospital in 1976 they found that 'the situation at Baragwanath was one patient under the bed, two in the bed and two on the floor.'[2]

The photographs in official South African publications do not show the mattresses on the floor, the infants two to a cot, or the casualty department littered with patients sleeping on the floor or on hard wooden benches. Those on the floor include the acutely ill and injured, as well as the less seriously ill patients. Because of the critical shortage of beds, over 13,000 patients are discharged each year before their treatment is complete, according to Dr. van der Heever, the Superintendent of Baragwanath.[3]

In 1983, doctors in the Department of Medicine at Baragwanath described the overcrowding and shortage of medical staff as having reached 'breaking point'. Journalists who visited Ward 21 found that its 40 beds were occupied by 89 women and one child. Red stickers marked 'Urgent' were stuck to the foreheads of critically ill patients and a doctor explained that 'we have to do that. It's the only way we can indicate the urgency of a case. There are not enough doctors and too many patients to do things any other way here.' Bedletters, giving the crucial medical and drugs history of each patient, often got lost in a confusion of movement as patients moved outside the wards during the day to give the doctors greater freedom to work inside. 'Sometimes I haven't been able to find out what medication a patient was receiving', one doctor said. 'People are not being treated properly here'.

At night, when the patients all moved back into the wards, more than half slept on the floor. Doctors and nurses attending the sick had to step over bodies packing the spaces between and under the beds. 'It is very hard for old grannies. If they have problems during the night we can't get to them easily. It is difficult to move', a nurse said.[4]

Similar conditions exist in other black hospitals. Coronation Hospital, which has only 505 beds, is supposed to serve the entire Coloured and Indian population of Johannesburg and the outlying areas, including Lenasia, the giant Indian ghetto situated 26 miles from the city centre. Lenasia has been in existence for 20 years and yet still has no hospital for its 65,000 residents. Although a number of doctors have taken it upon themselves to set up a 50-bed nursing home, few patients can afford the cost.

In Natal, the major hospital serving the entire black population of the province is King Edward VIII with 2,000 beds. King Edward Hospital deals with 600,000 out-patients a year and also has a bed occupancy of over 100 per cent.

Appalling conditions were reported in the maternity unit at the Livingstone Hospital in Port Elizabeth in 1977, with women in labour lying two to a bed, on mattresses on the floor and on trolleys in the corridors. Meanwhile, there were empty beds in the white section of the hospital.[5] Following the outcry, patients were accommodated in prefabricated buildings.

Five years and more later, pregnant women and those who had just given birth were still having to sleep two to a bed, or on the floor, at the Kalafong Hospital near Atteridgeville, Pretoria. Women in the maternity ward described it as a 'squatter area', and said that the majority of inmates were sleeping on the floor with the same blankets they used before giving birth. Others claimed that they had to use blankets dirtied by other patients who had been discharged.[6]

The administrative superintendent at Kalafong, Dr. J. A. Fourie, said that overcrowding was to blame, as it made it difficult to keep the hospital clean. There were 42 beds in the maternity section, but often double that number of patients. Dr. Fourie could not give statistics of the number of babies born daily at the hospital because of the fluctuation in the numbers of mothers-to-be.[7]

There were further complaints about discrimination and fees at Kalafong. A number of mothers-to-be complained about the lack and poor quality of the food provided and of 'exorbitant' fees following the introduction in April 1982 of a policy charging patients according to their salaries. One black businessman said that he had paid R300 for a 10 day stay at Kalafong, during which he had to sleep on the floor.[8] The chairman of the Atteridgeville Community Council said that the hospital was racially segregated and 'apartheid is very much alive there'. Black staff were refused permission to park their cars within the hospital grounds and the black women cleaning staff had to look after the white doctors' children.[9]

The story was similar at the Benoni-Boksburg Hospital when journalists went there in 1982 and 1983. Pregnant women were sleeping two or even three to a bed in the maternity ward, with others on the floor. One woman said that stout women were paired with slender ones in a desperate bid to make them 'comfortable'.[10] In the male surgical ward, again in the black section of the hospital, up to 90 patients slept on felt mats on the floor in a 32-bed ward. Meanwhile, 30 new wards were standing empty, and had been doing so for the past two years. Sources in the hospital said that the wards were originally intended as intensive care units for white patients, but the plan had to be abandoned because of a shortage of white nurses.[11]

In 1976, it was reported that at Groote Schuur Hospital in Cape Town (of heart transplant fame), black patients slept on trolleys, 'sometimes for weeks'. At the time, bed occupancy in the black section was 110 per cent and in the white section, 75 per cent.[12] During 1982, plans were set in motion to extend and develop Groote Schuur in a R200m building scheme, the largest ever undertaken by the Cape Provincial Administration. A completely new 1,440 bed hospital (300 more beds than the old) incorporating all the most modern ancillary treatment facilities was due to be built in the first, six year, phase, while overall, the 12 year redevelopment project was due to provide services for 10,000 people of all population groups daily.[13]

The huge scheme was criticised as a prestige project and a possible white elephant, going against world trends towards smaller hospitals and decentralised health services. Feeling was expressed that the authorities should instead be turning their attention to the lack of facilities in major

TABLE XX: Hospital beds, available and needed, 1983.

Population group	Beds available	Beds needed	
White	27,205	9,056	(18,112)
Black	43,935	40,716	(81,431)

Notes: The figures given for *available beds* exclude psychiatric beds for long term patients, TB beds and beds provided by mining and industry.

A breakdown of the beds available for black patients by population group is not available.

The first figures given for *beds needed* are calculated on the basis of two beds per 1,000 population (a ratio which assumes that 'all preventative measures are taken and adequate provision exists for primary health care'), and those in brackets on the basis of four beds per 1,000 population.

The figures exclude the 'independent' and 'self-governing' bantustans. The Minister noted that 'some of the beds for whites are interchangeable with those for non-whites'.

Source: Parliamentary reply from the Minister of Health and Welfare, *Debates,* 3.3.83.

growth areas such as Mitchells Plain, a Coloured township of nearly 150,000 people removed from other areas under the Group Areas Act. Mitchells Plain was served in 1983 by two polyclinics and three small day-hospitals run in converted houses. The Director of Provincial Hospital Services, Dr. R. L. M. Kotze, said that his department had originally been informed that the Mitchells Plain population (due to eventually reach 250,000) 'would be essentially middle-class, which usually generated its own private medical services. Nobody told us that a substantial section of the population would be on the sub-economic level.'[14]

In contrast to the overcrowded conditions in black hospitals white hospitals are not fully utilised. In Johannesburg, hospital facilities for whites include three hospitals, at least 15 private nursing homes, and a new R156 million, 2,000 bed hospital recently opened. This totals 4,000 beds. The average daily bed occupancy of the old white general hospital was only 69 per cent. Edenvale Hospital had 62 per cent occupancy and the J. G. Strijdom Hospital 77 per cent occupancy. While the Queen Victoria Maternity Unit for whites was due to be converted into residences for hospital maintenance staff because of underuse, Baragwanath had only 613 beds (including cribs) in the maternity units.[15]

Despite the extreme overcrowding at Baragwanath, it treats and admits a certain number of white patients as well as black — a fact cited by the authorities as evidence of a lack of discrimination in hospital services. During 1981, a total of about 200 white patients were treated at Baragwanath, mostly transferred from whites-only hospitals without particular facilities available at Baragwanath. Hospital authorities said that the practice of admitting whites had been going on since 1942 and the director of hospital services commented, 'why should it be illegal? There is no law that makes it illegal. We also treat Indians and Coloureds at the J. G. Strijdom Hospital. They are black and the hospital is white'. The report noted, however, that no black Africans were admitted to white hospitals in South Africa.[16]

In spite of the shortage of hospital beds for blacks, black hospitals are still being closed in the interests of rationalisation. A nutrition clinic for Africans at the Frere Hospital in the Eastern Cape was closed, for example, the patients being transferred to another hospital a 72 cents busfare away. This caused much hardship, as the patients, who were suffering from malnutrition anyway, were unable to afford the busfares. When asked about this, the director of hospital services replied that he was 'not there to give them busfares'.[17]

TABLE XXI: Hospitals and clinics in selected bantustans, 1981.

Bantustan	Number of clinics	Population per clinic	State hospitals Number	State hospitals Beds	Population[1] per hospital bed
Bophuthatswana[2]	119	12,000	n/a	4,528	n/a
Gazankulu	38	13,474	6[3]	1,517	338
KaNgwane	31	5,181	2	826	194
KwaNdebele	10	15,626	—	—	—
KwaZulu	130	26,217	26	7,935	400[4]
Lebowa	131	13,278	15	4,114	377[5]
QwaQwa	10	15,648	1	245	639
Transkei	175	17,000	n/a	n/a	n/a

n/a — figures not available.

Notes: 1. Also takes any private and mission hospitals into account.
2. The beds available in state hospitals in Bophuthatswana in 1981 broke down into general hospital beds — 2,493, psychiatric — 1,035 and tuberculosis — 1,000. The numbers of beds per 1,000 population were 1.8 (general hospitals), 0.8 (psychiatric) and 0.7 (tuberculosis).
3. Plus four day-hospitals with 16 beds each.
4. Also including three mission hospitals with a total of 586 beds.
5. Also including two private hospitals with a total of 500 beds.

Source: SAIRR, 1982, pp.540-1, citing figures published by the Bureau for Economic Research: Co-operation and Development (BENSO), the 1981 report of the Bophuthatswana Department of Health and Social Welfare and the 1982 report of the Transkei Department of Health.

Health services in the rural areas

The four 'independent' bantustans and all the 'self-governing' bantustans except KaNgwane and KwaNdebele have their own departments of health and welfare, which are responsible for the administration of the health services using funds allocated from each bantustan's budget.

In its *Survey of Race Relations* for 1982 the South African Institute of Race Relations, quoting a doctor who had written on the subject, noted that the bantustan health services

gave some credibility to the homeland administration itself by enabling it to promote services for local communities. The separation of rural health services into homeland health services allowed the government to manipulate health statistics to give the impression that the health status of SA's people was improving. An apparent fall in the rate of tuberculosis notifications between 1975 and 1980 was a result of the exclusion of statistics from Venda, Bophuthatswana and the Transkei. Dr. Zwi said that the separation of statistics also allowed the SA government to claim that most infectious diseases were occurring 'outside of SA' and were the responsibility of the appropriate homeland authority, not the SA Department of Health.[18]

From 1 April 1973, the Department of Bantu Administration and Development began a gradual takeover of all the mission hospitals. This was intended as an intermediate step, prior to handing over control and financing to the 'homeland governments'. Presented by the authorities as a 'progressive' move, the change has not improved services and has indeed created some additional problems. Mission hospitals under the control of Catholic missionaries were presented with a dilemma in that, under the government's health service scheme, hospitals receiving subsidies are obliged to provide advice and equipment for contraception. The takeover of the mission hospitals by the Department of Bantu Administration led to many resignations by doctors who did not wish to be under state control. Army doctors had to be called in to combat the resulting staff shortage. The takeover also resulted in some strange forms of hospital administration. For example the hospital of Umtata and Butterworth in the Transkei has two sections — the white section, which falls under the Department of Health of South Africa, and the black section which falls under the control of the Transkeian 'government'. (*See table XXI for statistics of hospitals and clinics in various bantustans, and Table XXII for statistics of medical personnel*). In some rural areas there is no primary care for the African community and patients have to travel long distances at great expense to obtain medical help.

The Natal provincial administration has spent about R26 million on a new hospital for whites in Pietermaritzburg to replace the existing hospital. By way of contrast, a hospital project started in Umlazi in 1968

69

TABLE XXII: Medical staff in selected bantustans, 1981.[1]

Bantustan	Medical & dental staff	Nursing staff	Paramedical staff	Pharmacists	Others[2]
Lebowa	95	1	13	12	5
Gazankulu	40	6	6	5	7
Venda	17	15	5	3	4
Ciskei	81	12	17	6	12
KwaZulu	265	23	28	21	184
QwaQwa	3	2	1	1	5
Bophuthatswana	90	46	8	7	20
Transkei	124	18	4	2	6

Notes: 1. The figures are of medical and paramedical personnel seconded to the bantustan health administrations.

2. Combines other professional staff, health inspectors, administrative, clerical, technical and auxiliary staff.

Source: SAIRR, 1982, p.541, citing figures extracted from the 1981 report of the Department of Health.

had, eight years later, proceeded no further than a few skeletal structures. When the question was raised in parliament the Minister replied that the hospital would be completed in 1981 subject to the availability of funds.[19]

The Garankua Hospital in Bophuthatswana, serving 60,000 people, is situated near Winterveld, a large, overcrowded and unhealthy resettlement area covered with squatters' shacks and lacking the most basic amenities. Garankua provides 14 clinics staffed by between two and six nurses, with a doctor visiting two to three times a week for an hour at a time. There is no electricity in the clinics and telephones are either non-existent or unreliable.

According to the 1981 annual report of the Bophuthatswana Department of Health and Social Welfare, there were a total of 81 doctors in the bantustan in 1981, 2,829 nurses and 2,135 medical staff of other ranks. There was one doctor per 17,000 population and one nurse per 500 population.[20]

In 1982, 'tens of thousands' of Transkeians were reported to be using the Natal provincial hospitals in Matatiele and Kokstad. Forty per cent of the Kokstad beds were said to be occupied by Transkeians and a spokesperson for the hospital board explained this was because the Transkei had 'no real health service'.[21]

Clinics

Many rural hospitals use the clinic or out-station to reach a large number of patients. In the more remote areas clinic staff may visit once a week, elsewhere they are in permanent attendance, able to refer serious cases to the hospital if necessary. This system is also used in the cities. Baragwanath Hospital has eight clinics attached to it. These are largely run by nursing staff with a doctor acting as consultant, trainer and monitor.**

In the Cape Town area, day hospitals, providing general and some specialised care on an out-patient basis are organised in a scheme designed to overcome the difficulties experienced by black residents in reaching medical services.[22]

The kind of discrimination encountered by black patients attending a clinic in Pretoria was described by a journalist from the black newspaper, *Sowetan*. Workers who became sick or were injured at work were referred to the clinic in Schoeman street, 'at the back of swank consulting rooms for whites', after treatment at Kalafong Hospital. While the white patients waited in a reception room furnished with sofas and magazines at the front of the premises, black patients had to wait under a small shelter round at the back made of four poles with a corrugated iron roof, and equipped with rough wooden benches. Others lay on the grass under the hot sun, during a wait of three hours or more to see the doctors.[23]

Hospital and clinic fees

Both blacks and whites are expected to pay for hospital and clinic treatment, although there are variations in the fees charged. Many whites are covered by insurance schemes.

During 1982, increased charges in government health services were announced. In April of that year, a new reclassification policy came into effect in most hospitals, under which patients were charged according to their incomes, and there were protests that in practice, this meant higher charges for the poor.[24] In the Transvaal, provincial hospital fees were doubled and in some cases trebled for the lowest income groups. Clinic and hospital fees for Africans who were not on any medical aid were increased from R1 to R2. Doctors in the Transvaal expressed the fear that increased fees might prevent chronically ill patients from returning for treatment.[25]

Five years earlier, in 1977, the Transvaal Administrator had announced an 80 per cent rise in hospital fees, saying that the contribution from patients' fees to hospital costs would rise from 8.3 per cent to 12.5 per cent. These increases bore particularly hard on black patients

---

**Footnote:* Black doctors withdrew their services from the clinics when their administration was taken over by the Transvaal Provincial Administration from the Johannesburg City Council. The takeover meant a drop in salaries. White doctors withdrew from the clinics after the Soweto uprising in June 1976.

as fees for full-paying black patients rose from R8 to R15 and for out-patients from R4 to R6. The cost of confinement for an African mother rose to R6 for residents in a proclaimed township (i.e. those permanently in the urban areas) and R12 for non-residents. Clinic fees in certain areas rose substantially so that in some income groups people not on medical aid paid more for a clinic visit than one to a private doctor.[26]

In a parliamentary debate in 1976 on tackling inflation in the health services, proposals made included reducing dosages of medicine by 25 per cent, charging 50 cents per patient for medical treatment given under relief services for the poor, requiring patients to contribute towards the cost of artificial aids and cutting down on staff and equipment.[27]

Health officials in South Africa stress the need for the private sector to play a greater role in the provision of health services, reflecting a new direction of state policy. The state's aim is to create a situation in which people pay for their own health care by using private doctors. This is disguised as 'self-help' and 'community development'.

In November 1982, it was announced that the first privately-owned black hospital in Southern Africa would be built the following year in Soweto. Described as a 'serious business venture', the hospital would cost R3,500,000. Dr. Nthato Motlana, director of the Lesedi Clinic, told journalists that a market survey conducted in early 1978 had shown that, at that time, Soweto could support a clinic of 250 beds for private patients. 'There are at present private nursing homes which do admit blacks', Dr. Motlana explained, 'but because of South Africa's strange racial laws these patients must be admitted to private wards with private toilets and baths — even separate cups and saucers.' He said that black patients were charged 'double what other races pay', which effectively put white nursing homes out of the reach of most of them.[28]

In the context of the health problems in Soweto, it is obvious that the proposed private black hospital will only have a limited impact. It is probably safe to assume that only a tiny minority will be able to afford to attend it.

Ambulance apartheid

Ambulances, like other branches of the health services, are racially segregated. Such segregation persists despite the higher costs entailed by duplicating the service between population groups, and the risks to patients themselves when refused admission to ambulances, and hospitals themselves, on racial grounds.

Incidents of 'ambulance apartheid' are described from time to time in the South African and overseas press. A particularly graphic account by a recent immigrant from Britain to South Africa was published in February 1983, for example:

72

Walking home late at night through Hillbrow, Johannesburg, I came across a young white man dying from stab wounds.

A black caretaker from a nearby block of flats was gently tending him.

Alarmed by the ghastly wounds, I dashed to the nearest phone to call an ambulance.

'Is he white?' inquired the woman with an Afrikaans accent on the end of the line.

'The man is dying. What difference does his colour make?'

'It depends which hospital we send an ambulance from,' the woman replied.

It shouldn't have shocked me — this is South Africa — but the cold face of apartheid *in extremis* chilled me into submission.

I said the man was white and put the phone down.

While waiting for the ambulance, I hailed a passing taxi and asked the driver to take the man to hospital.

'What's the matter with him?' asked the Portuguese driver.

'Two burglars stabbed him repeatedly in the face and neck with a screwdriver,' I said.

'Oh, he'll only get blood on my new seat covers.'

'But, for heaven's sake, the man is dying.'

'What colour is he?' the driver asked reluctantly.

At that moment the ambulance arrived, ending this spirited debate on the Christian ethics of separate development.

The ambulance had taken just four minutes, and the stabbed man's life was saved.

Had he been black, an ambulance would have had to come from further away, lengthening the time of the journey and the odds on his survival.[29]

Racial segregation in the health services means that patients often have to travel long distances to the nearest hospital catering for their population group. Some deaths inevitably result from the delays in initiating treatment. In theory, ambulance drivers are supposed to exercise their discretion in these matters, but in practice this seldom seems to happen. It is normal procedure for a driver to ascertain the population group of an injured person before setting out with an ambulance in response to an emergency call.

In July 1983, a nine-year-old African boy with serious head injuries resulting from a fall from the back of a farm lorry died after being refused admission to a hospital reserved for Indians. Zulinkosi Lindedu was taken to Northdale Hospital, north of Pietermaritzburg, after the accident on a nearby farm. He was refused admission and the farmer — himself an Indian — was told to take him to Edenvale Hospital, six miles away in the Kwazulu bantustan. The Northdale medical superintendent explained that the hospital was not allowed to admit Africans except in cases of 'extreme emergency'. Zulinkosi had seemed to be in a 'stable condition'.[30]

Zulinkosi was taken to Edenvale in the farmer's pick-up truck rather than an ambulance because, as a Northdale doctor explained, 'it would have taken much longer to get an ambulance here than it takes to get from here to Edenvale by car'. In the course of the journey, according to the farmer's son, the child went into a fit, and when he arrived at Edenvale was diagnosed as being in a critical condition. A white doctor ordered him to be transferred to Wentworth Hospital, Durban, 50 miles away, where there was a neurosurgical unit. Zulinkosi died the next day.[31]

In August 1982, a month-long investigation in Balfour, south-east of Johannesburg, exonerated the town's ambulance service from any blame after an incident in which a black worker lay bleeding for five hours before being taken to hospital. The patient, Johan Botha, was given emergency treatment by a local doctor for serious open wounds caused by a drum of thinners exploding at the glass factory where he worked. The doctor then tried to arrange admission to hospital, but found that Balfour's black ambulance service was out of town. The company refused to allow Botha to be taken to hospital by car and eventually, after delay, an ambulance from a meat factory was used.[32]

In 1983, the Jabulani Ambulance and Fire Department revealed that only four ambulances were available at weekends to cater for the inhabitants of Soweto. Dr. Nthato Motlana, the chairman of the Soweto Committee of Ten, commented that the ambulance drivers tended to operate like buses, picking up casualties throughout Soweto regardless of the fact that their passengers included serious cases needing immediate attention.[33]

Official concern over ambulance apartheid is usually concern for delays affecting white patients. Parity between the salaries of white and Coloured ambulance drivers was introduced in the Cape peninsula to try to eliminate this problem.

Non-emergency ambulance services are generally expensive and far beyond the means of many blacks. In 1979 the fees were R10 to R15 payable in cash.[34] In the rural areas, in consequence, sick patients often end up walking miles for medical treatment.

In October 1982 the Johannesburg *Sunday Times* published a letter from a middle-aged woman, describing an incident outside a hotel in Maritzburg. The writer and her sister had gone to the aid of an African man trapped beneath a car. 'I tried to get the white men around to lift the car off the man', she said. 'They were disinclined to do so — many holding glasses in their hands. One told me: "Leave him, he smells . . ." The man was indeed grimy as well as being covered in blood.

'One man finally helped me and we lifted him onto the pavement while laughter rang out from the balcony of the hotel. I was told that the manager of the hotel had not phoned for an ambulance but had "lodged a complaint with the police" about the incident.' When the man was finally taken away in an ambulance the two women were told they would have to pay for this service.[35]

Blood transfusions and heart transplants

There is in South Africa legislation requiring that the population group of the blood donor should be stipulated on every container of human blood. There is, however, no prohibition of inter-racial blood transfusion.[36]

This practice of labelling blood according to population group persists in South Africa, despite evidence that there is no racial difference in blood. Research carried out by the Human Serum Genetics Unit, South African Institute for Medical Research, Johannesburg, showed that 'there appears to be no good serogenetic reason for the labelling of containers of human blood with the race of the donor'.[37]

Blood from black donors is not used for white patients in South Africa, however, although blood from white donors is used for black patients. This was confirmed by the South African Blood Transfusion Service in January 1984. The deputy director of the South African Department of Health, explained that it was the 'custom' in South Africa to use blood donated by black people mainly for black patients because of what he described as 'practical, scientific reasons' arising out of the higher incidence of hepatitis among black people. To justify the transfusing of possibly contaminated hepatitis B virus blood to black patients, he explained that black people *might* have a greater immunity to the disease as a result of exposure to the same antigens. In reply, a spokesman for the National Medical and Dental Association commented: 'The implication of this is that it is alright for black people to be infected by the hepatitis virus but not for other race groups to be affected'.[38] It has not been explained why the risk of hepatitis infection from transfusion could not be avoided by screening as has been done in other countries.

It is interesting to note that there are no such qualms when it comes to providing black donor organs for white patients. In August 1982, a Cape Town surgeon found himself at the centre of a controversy when he told the Transplantation Society's international congress in Brighton, England, that patients with transplant hearts from black donors survived nearly three times longer than those with hearts from white donors. Dr. David Cooper, an English immigrant who in 1982 was running Professor Christian Barnard's pioneering heart transplant unit at Groote Schuur Hospital, also said that hearts from African donors were significantly better than those from Coloured donors. 'This is the sort of data you have to handle very carefully in South Africa', he added.

Dr. Cooper later said that he had been quoted out of context by the London *Guardian*, and that his address to the Transplantation Society had been reported in an 'unbalanced way'. The work at the Groote Schuur unit would go ahead without change: 'There is a great shortage of donors, and we will take any heart we can get for our patients', Dr. Cooper said.[39]

Blood donors are also in short supply in South Africa. In 1982, a spokesman for the Blood Transfusion Services in Johannesburg indicated that one reason was a belief among black people that any blood they gave would be used to 'save the government's military men at the border.'[40]

Medical aid schemes

Health insurance or medical schemes expanded rapidly in South Africa after World War II, and by 1978 a total of 254 separate schemes had been registered.[41] The schemes, which are financed by both employer and employee, fall into two main groups: medical benefit, or assistance, schemes, and medical aid schemes. Medical aid schemes are aimed at the skilled, higher-paid workers and the benefits are more extensive than those under the medical benefit schemes.

Although black membership of medical schemes has increased more rapidly than white, the percentage of the black population covered by such health insurance is still very small. By 1977, 76 per cent of the white population were beneficiaries of medical schemes (i.e. members and their dependants), but only 3.4 per cent of blacks. Overall, only 16.4 per cent of the South African population were covered by medical schemes.[42]

This racial discrepancy has resulted from the primary application of the schemes to skilled workers and the size of the contributions required, which are too high for the lower paid workers. Furthermore, existing medical aid schemes for blacks tend to cover ordinary consultations and medicines only, whereas whites are covered for all treatment. In effect the black worker is subsidising his or her white counterpart.

In 1978 a group of black doctors and businessmen in Johannesburg launched a new medical aid scheme for blacks. The contributions were small enough for most workers to be able to pay on a 50-50 basis with their employers and the fund scheme became known as the Sizwe (*The Nation*) Medical Aid Fund. One of the members of the board, Dr. Nthato Motlana, was unable to attend the launching of the scheme as he had just entered his sixth month of detention without trial.[43] By the end of 1982, the Sizwe Medical Aid Fund had a membership of over 6,000 and cash reserves of over R400,000.[44]

A clinic started in Paarl by two trade unions for workers in canning factories is another example of medical self-help and is believed in South Africa to be the first of its kind on the continent. The African Food and Canning Workers Union (AFCWU) and the Food and Canning Workers Union (FCWU) set up the clinic in 1981 under the auspices of their medical fund (the Fruit and Vegetable Canning Workers Medical Benefit Fund) out of concern that large amounts of money were passing into the hands of private doctors. Instead of *pro rata* payments to the latter, the Paarl clinic was in 1983 buying medicines in bulk and dispensing them free to workers. The fund was maintained through weekly deductions from workers' salaries and contributions from management, entitling the workers to attend the clinic as often as required. The cost to the clinic of medicines per worker averaged out at R1.40, compared with R5 — R10 per worker being paid out by the union's medical fund in other parts of the country.[45]

Welfare services and social security

All social and welfare services are segregated by population group, the provisions for white people being again far superior to those for black.

In the 1982-83 budget, more than twice as much was allocated for the care of elderly white people as for African, despite the much greater numerical size of the African population. The exact figures, which included provision for old age and veterans' pensions, were as follows:

White	R295,761,600
African	R129,571,000
Indian	R20,613,300
Coloured	R104,660,600[46]

In 1981 there were a total of 426 old age homes for elderly white people, comprising four state homes, 334 subsidised homes and 88 non-subsidised homes. One state home had been provided for Coloured people, together with 25 private registered homes, run by welfare societies and churches. For African elderly, only seven private homes existed, accommodating a total of 283 people, while temporary care for 102 people was provided by administration boards at three centres. In addition, five homes existed in the 'self-governing' bantustans, together with 493 'places' (unspecified) for the elderly.[47]

Only two homes existed in 1981 for Indian elderly, both private registered.[48] One in Durban accommodated 743 persons in 1976, while the other in Pietermaritzburg, run by the Asian Benevolent Society, accommodated 10 persons.[49]

In 1982, the percentage of white South Africans living in state-subsidised and private old-age homes was reported to be the highest in the world — 28,000 people or 11 per cent of the population over the age of 65.[50]

There is no national social security scheme in South Africa. In 1979-80 a total of 199,565 African people in the 'white' areas were receiving old age pensions, compared to 141,154 white, 19,003 Indian and 90,164 Coloured. In addition, a total of 367,018 African elderly were, in 1980-81, receiving old age pensions in the 'self-governing' bantustans.[51] To be eligible for such a pension, an aged African must have an income of less than R80 per annum and assets not exceeding R2,450. The number of aged Africans who would be disqualified by such a means test is very small indeed, yet it is clear that many old people fail to receive their pension benefits. In 1977 it was reported that in the Grahamstown area 300 Africans lost their pensions and a further 358 were due to suffer a similar fate because they were unable to furnish acceptable proof of their dates of birth. (Such a dilemma is hardly surprising considering that it has not been compulsory for Africans to register births and deaths). The pension they should have received was a mere R15 per month.[52]

The pension rates vary according to population group. Social pensions (i.e. old age, disability, blind persons and veterans' pensions) were increased with effect from 1 October 1982. The rates from then were as follows:

	White	Indian/Coloured	African
Maximum monthly amount payable (R)	138	83	49
increase (R)	16	12	9[53]

African pensioners are paid every second month, presumably for administrative convenience. Long queues at pay-out points and long delays in processing applications are common. In the bantustan areas, where elderly relatives often have to care for children while their parents work in the cities, such pensions may be the sole income for a household of several people.

In 1982, a scheme was set in motion in Soweto to try and improve conditions at the pay-out points established in the huge township for more than 22,000 pensioners. Many pensioners were crippled and infirm, yet they arrived early in the morning, irrespective of the weather, to join the open-air queues. The Paballo Soweto Pensioners' Pay-Out Ministry, a body with church connections, was reportedly planning to set up soup kitchens at the pay-out points, and to help with transport and other services for pensioners.[54]

78

In March 1983 the South African government announced a R100 million increase for pensioners, including a one-off R29 million bonus, to be paid out in May. Social pensions for white people would rise by R14 a month with effect from 1 October 1983, to R152; by R10 a month for Coloured and Indian, to R93; and by R8 a month for African, to R57. The maximum assets limit for white social pensioners would be raised from R34,800 to R42,000 and the maximum annual income limit from R1,393 to R1,920. Existing means test ratios for Coloured, Indian and African pensioners, however, would remain in force.[55]

Children's homes

The problem of neglected and abandoned children in South Africa is a serious one due to the migrant labour system, influx control laws, poverty and poor living conditions. In 1979 it was reported that the Johannesburg Welfare Society was taking two children into its care every day, on average, after they had been abandoned in Soweto.[56]

Provision for needy black children is grossly inadequate. The 1982-83 budget allocated R6,240,000 for African child welfare, R64,497,300 for white children, R26,147,700 for Indian and R84,467,100 (the highest figure) for Coloured.[57]

In 1981, there were seven state places of safety and detention and 80 private registered children's homes for whites, caring for a total of 6,950 children. A total of 23,056 African children in 'white' areas were cared for in 191 registered places of care, five privately-controlled children's homes and six places of safety, four of which were state institutions.[58]

The *per capita* monthly maintenance grants available for children in welfare homes vary according to population group, with a maximum of R150.80, or the actual cost at a particular home, whichever is the lesser amount, being allocated for white children and R40 for African (1982 figures).[59]

There is only one home for Coloured children in the Transvaal and Orange Free State — the St. Joseph's Home in Johannesburg. Twenty-five per cent of the inmates are there because of illegitimacy or because they have been classified as racially different from their parents. A child with mixed parentage is discouraged from applying to be classified as 'white' because '. . . it is claimed their own children will face the same problem all over again.'[60]

In 1981 there was one state home for 174 Coloured children and 23 private registered homes which cared for 1,803 children. There were six homes for Indian children, with places for 384 children. The monthly *per capita* maintenance grant for Indian and Coloured children in welfare homes in 1982 was R100.64 or the actual cost of a particular home, whichever was the lesser.[61]

Foster care grants for children from the different racial categories also vary sharply. In 1982 the grants were R90, R61 and R24 a month for white, Coloured, Indian and African children respectively.[62]

Because of the inadequate provision for needy black children, in most of the major cities it is not uncommon to find bands of apparently homeless youngsters sleeping rough and living by casual labour, begging and scavenging. The state does little to provide remedial child care, the bulk of child welfare work being undertaken by autonomous black organisations. The major burden tends to be borne by relatives.[63]

Physical disability

In a country where health and social services for the physically 'normal' black citizen are distinctly inferior to the facilities provided for whites, it comes as no surprise to discover that facilities for physically disabled black people are practically non-existent.

The following amounts were allocated to welfare services for the disabled in the 1982/83 budget:

	1982/83	1981/82	
White	R5,769,000	R5,251,400	
Indian	R81,000	Not available	
Coloured	R305,000	Not available	
African	R527,000	R537,700	[64]

Africans, comprising 72.7 per cent of the population, were allocated less than one tenth of the amount allocated to the whites, comprising 15.5 per cent of the population.

Details of institutions for the disabled extracted from departmental reports reveal that in 1981 there were a total of 40 institutions for whites as well as protective workshops. For handicapped Coloured people there were only seven workshops, subsidised by the Department of Internal Affairs. The only institution for African cerebral palsied subsidized by the department in 1980/81 was at Madadeni. This accommodated 80 children.[65]

Blind persons may be admitted to workshops for the blind in the bantustans or to two institutions in Port Elizabeth and Kimberley. The following facilities for the disabled were available in the 'self governing' bantustans:

Institutions for the cerebral palsied — one in Gazankulu housing 250 people.

Institutions for the blind and deaf — one in Gazankulu for 80 people; one in QwaQwa for 120 people.

80

Handicraft centres — one in Kwazulu for 80 people; one in QwaQwa for 108 people; two in Gazankulu for 53 people.

Institutions for the physically handicapped — three in Kwazulu for 350 people; one in QwaQwa for 97 people; three in Lebowa for 280 people.[66]

In 1982 it was reported that the South African government had contributed R1 million towards the cost of a sports complex for the physically disabled in Soweto. The full estimated cost of the complex was R3.5 million.

In reality, the original plan for the complex had not been conceived by any state department but by an enterprising individual, Mr. Mavuso, who, though innocent, had been shot and crippled for life by a police bullet. While in hospital he had witnessed the plight of other physically disabled patients, who after discharge from hospital, found themselves back in the wards some months later suffering from bed sores, infections and poor nutrition. This situation reflected the lack of facilities outside of the hospital for the care of the disabled, and the inadequacy of their disability grants of R40 per month for providing rent, food and transport.

Through the personal initiative of Mr. Mavuso, joint meetings between patients and staff at the hospital were arranged and a fund started. The original enterprise was short-lived as the hospital authorities banned the meetings because they did not wish to have business ventures discussed on hospital premises. After years of begging for funds, a meeting between Mr. Mavuso and the South African Sports Association for the Physically Disabled finally got things moving through a government grant of R1 million.

Soweto accommodates about 500 paraplegics, the largest concentration of physically disabled people in South Africa. Their disabilities are in most cases the results of assaults by knives, bicycle spokes and gunshot wounds. They have an abnormally high mortality rate because of pressure sores and bladder and kidney infections leading to kidney failure, particularly in those who lack sensation in the lower halves of their bodies. An organisation called the Soweto Self-Help Association of Paraplegics (SHAPS), formed by Mr. Mavuso and his colleagues, found that most paraplegics were not properly informed by hospitals of how their condition would change their bodily functions. It was only through the initiative of SHAPS that two paraplegics were trained to lecture to others on health care.

The high mortality rate among African paraplegics in Soweto is also a reflection of the poor and overcrowded living conditions for the average Sowetan. It is difficult to accommodate a person in a wheelchair in a tiny house which may be crammed with 10 or even 20 people. Paraplegics, 70 per cent of whom are unemployed in Soweto, are a burden on families already struggling to feed their children. Most paraplegics in Soweto lose their rights to their homes at the same time as losing their jobs on becoming disabled. They have to become lodgers, usually at exorbitant rents. Houses with special facilities for wheelchairs are unheard of. SHAPS has also taken on the task of trying to find employment for its members.[67]

In most cases the State provides only part of the funds required for facilities for the physically disabled, usually the running costs. The actual establishment of special workshops, schools and clinics has usually been the result of work done by charitable institutions and has been funded by public donations. A R250,000 project to build workshops, schools and clinics in the Austerville area, near Durban, for about 60 disabled Coloured adults, for example, was initiated by the Natal Association for the Care of the Coloured Physically Disabled. The money for the project was raised by public contributions and charitable institutions, and part of the sum required was borrowed as a 'soft' loan. Ninety five per cent of the running costs were due to be paid by the State.[68]

Similarly, in Pinetown, also near Durban, a R3 million school for 300 physically handicapped black children (of whom there were reported to be more than 2,000 in the greater Durban area alone) was due to be built at the end of 1982. The establishment of this school was initiated by the Pinetown Central Rotary Club, which later handed the funding to a committee, the Ethembeni Association. A government grant would provide 95 per cent of the running costs.[69]

In Soweto, a total of two houses have been made available to old and disabled people by the West Rand Administration Board. Aided by a charitable organisation, the Housewives League, they have provided furniture and made regular donations of food and old clothing. Clearly, in a town like Soweto, with a population conservatively estimated at one million people, this is quite inadequate to deal with the problems faced by the elderly disabled.

In 1982, it was reported that those disabled workers who had jobs were in danger of losing them, because the Cripple Care Association which provided transport to and from their work lacked sufficient funds and vehicles to carry on the service. Although the Association's disabled passengers contributed to the costs if they could afford it, there was no subsidy to meet the running expenses. A decline in the donations on which the Association relied, coupled with rising costs, had forced it to curtail its activities.[70]

Health care for blind black people, especially in the rural areas, is for practical purposes non-existent except for services provided by a mobile eye clinic established in 1981 by the South African Bureau for the Prevention of Blindness. In 1983 this operated in the Kwazulu, Transkei, Venda, Lebowa, QwaQwa and Bophuthatswana bantustans, where it made five three-day visits a year. The Bureau owned two other mobile clinics which made infrequent visits while one was operational in Namibia. A group of about 30 ophthalmologists in the country operated permanently in the rural areas.[71]

The only eye clinic outside of a hospital in South Africa was opened in March 1983 by the Natal African Blind Society in Umlazi near Durban. The clinic is funded by donations and charitable organisations and technical staff work there on a voluntary basis.[72]

Information about facilities for the black deaf is difficult to find. The South African National Council for the Deaf, founded in 1929, provides facilities for 2,000 people through 236 social workers and has 3,000 children at schools for the deaf — all of them white. An estimated 7,000 white people in South Africa are 'prelingual' deaf (i.e. deaf from birth) but no figures are available for blacks. It appears as if deaf black people are not considered in the Council's reckoning at all.[73]

During 1983 the South African National Council for the Deaf was engaged in negotiations for readmission to the World Sport Federation of the Deaf, with a view to taking part in the Olympic Silent Games in Los Angeles in 1985. It might not be surprising in the light of South Africa's need for favourable international publicity if facilities for the black deaf inside the country were improved.

Summary

The segregation of medical and social services according to population group in South Africa is unique in the world. The incredible misuse of money and resources that results from the duplication of health services can only be explained by the apartheid need to maintain discrimination in both the quantity and the quality of the health and welfare services provided for whites and for blacks.

Whites, the minority group, enjoy the best and most plentiful supply of health care. Their health facilities are in fact underutilized, resulting in empty beds or even the actual closure of some white hospitals, while those for blacks are over-crowded and understaffed. The major hospitals, furthermore, are all situated in the urban areas, while the rural areas — those of greatest need — are deprived of readily available and adequate health facilities.

8. Health Workers

White South Africans enjoy easy access to doctors and other qualified health personnel.

At the end of 1981, a total of 3,920 medical specialists and 16,787 general medical practitioners were registered with the South African Medical and Dental Council. Although an official breakdown of these figures by population group was not available, a South African medical expert estimated that the doctor:patient ratio was 1:330 for white people, 1:730 for Indian, 1:12,000 for Coloured and 1:91,000 for African. Overall, the ratio was 1:1,540, excluding the bantustans of Transkei, Bophuthatswana and Venda.[1] (In practice many white doctors do serve black patients — see below).

This estimate of 1:91,000 for the African population compares unfavourably with figures cited by the South African Department of Information itself for a number of other African countries, for the years 1973-74. The ratio for Angola, for example, was given as 1:15,400, 1:10,480 (Botswana), 1:25,460 (Nigeria) and 1:59,600 (Upper Volta).[2]

Other sources have estimated that in the mid-1970s, at least 93 per cent of medical practitioners in South Africa were white.[3] The doctor:patient ratios for South Africa do not directly reflect the availability of health care for the different groups as many blacks are treated by white personnel, but they do reflect the discrepancies in the availability of facilities for medical training. Similar discrepancies occur in the figures for nurses and other medical personnel.

The distribution of doctors

Medical practitioners are also very unequally distributed geographically. While approximately 60 per cent of the population live in rural areas, only five per cent of doctors practise there.[4] In the urban areas, medical practitioners are further concentrated in white residential and business districts.[5]

The distribution of doctors by university of training also illustrates the bias of skills and expertise, including specialist skills, towards the urban areas. In the rural areas 30 per cent of all doctors are from non-South African universities, reflecting the high proportion of ex-mission hospitals in the rural areas, often staffed by overseas personnel.

The universal trend towards specialisation has affected South African medical training which is now geared towards producing doctors who are highly trained in the field of diagnostic and curative medicine. Between 1946 and 1976, the number of specialists as a percentage of all doctors in South Africa rose from 13.6 to 24.6 per cent. Preventative medicine tends to be ignored or to receive minimal attention. Until recently the University of Cape Town did not even have a department of preventative medicine. Public health is not a popular field either.[6]

Emigration also affects the provision of medical care. In the six years 1970-75 inclusive (quiet years politically in South Africa) it is estimated that 14 per cent of all medical graduates left the country permanently. Since then, emigration by doctors from South Africa for financial and political reasons has continued, causing great concern.[7] A total of 123 doctors are officially recorded as having left South Africa permanently in 1979, 59 in 1980 and 55 in 1981 (preliminary estimate).[8]

Medical training

The vast majority of medical students in South Africa are white, just as the medical profession as a whole is heavily white-dominated (*see Table XXIII*). Medical education for whites is provided at the universities of Pretoria, Cape Town, Witwatersrand, Orange Free State and Stellenbosch. Small numbers of black students have in the past been able to train at three 'open' universities for medical studies, namely Cape Town, Witwatersrand and Natal. There are no separate centres for the training of Coloured and Indian doctors. In 1978, special provision was made for African students through the establishment of Medunsa (Medical University of South Africa), a medical school at Garankua in the Bophuthatswana bantustan. This is actually part of a plan to phase them out of the other centres of training.

Up until the late 1970s most African medical students were trained at the University of Natal Medical School. This was opened in 1951 and was for black students. In 1966, new regulations were introduced under the ineptly-named Extension of University Education Act of 1959, requiring black medical students who wished to train at the alternative venues of the University of the Witwatersrand and Cape Town to obtain special ministerial dispensation first. The Extension of University Education Act was designed to close the 'mixed' universities to black students. Ministerial permission was more easily granted to Indian and Coloured students than to African. In 1978, 82.9 per cent of Indian and 95.2 per cent of Coloured applicants were granted permission, but only 29.1 per cent of African.

Up to the end of 1971 a total of only 252 African doctors had been trained, all of them at the universities of Natal and Witwatersrand. A report in 1969 quoted the Director of Hospital Services as saying that the ban on admitting African students to Witwatersrand Medical School had been 'slightly' lifted in order to allow African doctors to train as specialists.[9]

TABLE XXIII: Acceptance to medical schools for the first year course in 1981.

University	White	African	Indian	Coloured	Chinese
Pretoria	220	—	—	—	—
Witwatersrand	179	15	9	8	6
Orange Free State	118	—	—	—	—
Cape Town	147	—	6	17	—
Natal	—	30	39	—	—
Stellenbosch	160	—	—	4	—
Medunsa	—	40	—	5	—
Total	824	85	54	34	6

Source: SAIRR, 1982, p.546 (citing figures given in parliament).

In 1975 the Natal Medical School became a casualty of the government plan to remove all African students from white universities. On 17 December 1975 the Department of National (white) Education informed the Faculty of Medicine at Natal University that no more African students were to be admitted. Following a protest strike by the students it was agreed to admit African students for one more year but to enforce the exclusion order from 1978. After further discussions between the Minister of Education and the university authorities the government again temporarily postponed its decision, but one of the reasons for their retreat was that the new medical school at Garankua was not yet ready to open. The school is now functioning and is intended to provide medical, dental, and veterinary training for Africans; it is under the Minister of Education and Training (formerly Bantu Education), who has the power to vet all applicants. In 1981, Medunsa had a total of 578 students in medical and paramedical faculties.[10] Its first graduation ceremony was due to be held at the end of November 1982.[11]

The government is also planning to set up a medical school for Indian students only at the University of Durban-Westville (one of the 'bush' colleges established to keep blacks out of the white universities). This was announced by the Minister at the opening of the third session of the South African Indian Council in Durban in November 1974. To this end a professor of anatomy had already been appointed.[12] In 1976 it was announced that the government had also made a decision to phase out Coloured and Indian students of medicine from the University of Cape Town.[13]

White people, who represented less than one fifth of the total population over the years 1968-77, comprised 88.4 per cent of all new doctors trained during this period, while the African group, comprising 70.4 per cent of the total population, produced only three per cent of all doctors in this period. In other words, the white population produced 98 doctors per one million white citizens, while the African produced *one* doctor per *two* million of its population. The output of all black doctors remained virtually unchanged from four per million in 1967 to 4.8 per million in 1975,[14] while the output of white doctors increased from 92 to 142 per million whites.

The policy of limiting the number of admissions is part of the overall strategy of 'Bantu Education'. As Dr. Verwoerd put it in 1954: 'There is no place for him (the Bantu) in the European community above the level of certain forms of labour . . . Until now he has been subjected to a school system which drew him away from his own community and misled him by showing him the green pastures of European society in which he is not allowed to graze.'[15] The Report of the Departmental Committee on Native Education (1935-36) summed up the policy as follows: 'The education of the white child prepares him for life in a dominant society and the education of the black child for a subordinate society . . . The limits (of Native Education) form part of the social and economic structure of the country.'[16]

TABLE XXIV: Medical students qualifying as doctors at the end of 1980.

University	White	African	Indian	Coloured
Pretoria	169	—	—	—
Witwatersrand	176	4	7	4
Orange Free State	61	—	—	—
Cape Town	137	—	7	14
Natal	—	47	48	—
Stellenbosch	114	—	—	—
Total	657	51	62	18

The first 38 medical students graduated from Medunsa in November 1982. The Minister of Education and Training stated that 34 had qualified as doctors.

Source: SAIRR, 1982, p.546; *Debates* 3.3.83.

This policy is entrenched in the laws of the country which have made education compulsory for whites but not for blacks. Whereas blacks have to pay towards their education, including the cost of books and stationery, whites do not. The central government and provincial administrations were due to spend 61 per cent of the total educational budget for 1982-83 on white education compared to 17.7 per cent on African education.[17] The rest of the expenditure required for African education comes out of the pockets of the African people themselves in the form of taxes, levies and donations. The *per capita* expenditure during 1981-82 on African school pupils was less than one seventh that on whites (R165.23 compared to R1,221).[18]

Poor educational provision for African children is reflected in the figures for university enrolment which despite increases over the years show a basic racial imbalance.

Discrimination in access to facilities occurs within the so-called 'mixed' universities. At the Medical Faculty at the University of the Witwatersrand, for example, black students are barred from attending post mortems on whites. In one year an attempt was made to 'ease' the situation by allowing black students into the post mortem room after the organs had been removed and the corpse covered up. At the University of Cape Town black students are not allowed to attend post mortems on whites, but the mortuary attendants are black.

During the clinical years of training, black students are not allowed to attend ward rounds in white hospitals, nor are they allowed to examine white patients. White students attend ward rounds at both white and black hospitals and are free to examine all patients. The result is that white students receive a better all-round education. Furthermore it is accepted practice for white students to gain experience on black patients before undertaking the same procedures on whites. For the same reason many white doctors elect to do their early years in medical practice in black hospitals to obtain the necessary skill and expertise before entering practice in white hospitals. This is also true of doctors from abroad who come to South Africa to obtain experience.

Because most professorial units are situated in the white hospitals, black students almost never get the chance to attend professorial ward rounds. Discrimination also affects their attendance at lectures held at white hospitals. Black students may be asked to leave the lecture theatre if white patients are to be brought in for clinical demonstrations.

Discrimination affects black doctors when they have qualified and find themselves overlooked for promotion. Many find white registrars who have actually been trained under their own tutorship and guidance, being promoted above their heads. This was particularly noticeable at the medical school in Natal University, which, being exclusively for black students, might have been expected to appoint black people to professorial positions. However, when the professorial post in obstetrics and gynaecology fell vacant, one of the white registrars who had trained under an African consultant in obstetrics and gynaecology was given the position, rather than the consultant himself. In replying to a press article exposing the decision, Professor Smythe, Dean of the Faculty of

Medicine, said that 'there was nothing wrong in the appointment of a white gynaecologist who was junior in service to a more experienced black doctor'. He went on to explain that it was only a temporary measure. Incidentally, the white doctor in question had been qualified in the speciality for 17 months, the black doctor for 10 years.[19] Subsequently a white professor was imported from Salisbury, Rhodesia (now Harare, Zimbabwe) and the black consultant in question finally accepted a post as professor at the new medical school for Africans at Garankua.

In recent years a few Indian doctors in Durban have been given professorial posts, probably with the new Indian medical school in mind. One of the main reasons given for not appointing black doctors to professorial posts is that they would then be in a position of authority over white doctors.

Doctors' salaries

After a long struggle, including strike action, black doctors have attained parity in salaries with white doctors. Parity has still not been reached, however, in the grade of Medical Officer, while the Minister, in citing the figures, did not give the scale for interns. This means that, in practice, most black doctors, who are usually not specialists, are still being paid less than their white counterparts.

Apart from salary discrimination black doctors also face poor promotion prospects, differences in annual and sick leave, poor accommodation (four doctors sharing one room with one telephone when on night duty, for example), no married quarters or travel allowances (only provided for whites), and poor recreation facilities.

Some white consultants at Baragwanath were reported to practise discrimination in never employing black housemen in their wards. Instead, the posts were given to whites, who had a choice of many hospitals in which to work, while blacks only had a choice of two. The first black doctor to become head of a medical unit at Baragwanath was appointed in 1974.[20]

In the past, black doctors were not allowed to examine white patients in provincial hospitals although many black doctors saw white patients in their private practices. However, in 1976 it was decided that if a white patient wished to see a black doctor in a provincial hospital, the case would be assessed on its merits. This change occurred when a number of white patients at the Addington Hospital in Durban required the expertise of some of the black consultants at King Edward VIII Hospital. In another case an Indian doctor was barred from assisting in an operation on a white child who had been his patient for three years. The Natal Director of Hospital Services, Dr. W. Botha, subsequently stated that if white patients wished to be treated by black doctors they could go to black hospitals.[21]

If black patients wish to be admitted to private white hospitals, they require special permits from the Department of Community Development.[22]

According to one medical commentator, 'White South African nurses are unwilling to accept orders from a non-white doctor (except in a real emergency when no White doctor is available), in which they have the backing of their association, the public in general, and the present government.'[23]

Many members of the medical profession in South Africa approach their black patients as, in the first instance, objects of scientific interest. The Deputy Superintendent of Baragwanath Hospital, for example, described it as a 'disease palace', explaining that 'you can see a greater variety of diseases here in a short time than anywhere else in the world.'[24]

It is an unfortunate fact that doctors are often indifferent to black patients as human beings and see them simply as 'interesting cases'. Sometimes their behaviour is callous and indifferent. Patients are often shouted at, insulted or subjected to humiliating and degrading treatment. A black patient's dignity is seldom respected. Patients are examined in full view of everyone including casual cleaners in the ward.

Black women at a clinic in Edenvale in the Transvaal were reported to have been subjected to 'concentration camp treatment'. They were made to stand around in their underwear while a doctor performed vaginal examinations in full view of other patients waiting. There were also no curtains on the windows. When questioned about this, the doctor concerned, Dr. Theo Fairly, admitted that the allegations were basically correct, but said that he was 'progressive' and denied that he treated Africans 'like cattle'. He saw nothing wrong with his behaviour and said so. He claimed the women were not upset because they are 'black and natives are more communal and don't mind . . .'[25]

General practice in South Africa

Black doctors in general practice may only work in their own 'ethnic' group. In 1969, the then Department of Bantu Administration issued a circular to the effect that non-white doctors would no longer be granted consulting rooms and offices in urban areas, i.e. the African townships, because such communities were situated in 'white' areas.[26] White doctors cannot live in the African townships and this means that townships residents have no medical care at night or at weekends. Black doctors and 'other professional Africans' are supposed to work in the 'homelands'.[27]

In accordance with this ruling an African medical practitioner was refused permission to practise in Uitenhage near Port Elizabeth. At the time there were five non-resident doctors in New Brighton (the black township in the area) tending 150,000 inhabitants. Similarly, three Indian doctors were ordered out of their consulting rooms in an area proclaimed for whites. These doctors had been serving a population of 77,000 African and Coloured people. Similarly in Bergville and Mooi River 100,000 African patients were affected when two Indian doctors were disqualified from remaining in areas proclaimed as 'white' under the Group Areas Act (No.36/1966).[28]

Dentists and dental facilities

According to the South African Medical and Dental Council there were 2,794 dentists registered in South Africa as at 31 December 1981.[29] The dental service in South Africa has been described by the Minister of Health as being 'so inefficient, unbalanced, and unco-ordinated that [it fails] to meet the needs of the country.'[30]

TABLE XXV: Enrolled dental students, 1979-80.

University	White	Coloured	Indian	Chinese	African	Total	Qualified 1979
		1980 Enrolment					
Pretoria	359	—	—	—	—	359	61
Stellenbosch	289	—	—	—	—	289	41
Western Cape	—	34	56	—	—	90	14
Witwatersrand	294	1	10	6	6	317	43
Total	942	35	66	6	6	1,055	159

Source: SAIRR, 1980, p.574.

Dental training for blacks is of relatively recent date as existing dental schools were previously barred to them. By 1968 only one African dentist had been trained in South Africa.[31] In 1973 a dental school was established at the University of the Western Cape for Coloured students but by 1980 there were still only 50 black dentists and dental therapists.[32]

The provincial authorities provide dental services for white school children only and there are no provisions for Africans. In the bantustans there are nine clinics with full time dentists. The dental school at the University of the Witwatersrand provides a 'service', but patients have to wait up to six months for an appointment.

At clinics dental services are provided by nurses, who, not being trained in dentistry, simply perform extractions. This often occurs in dental departments at busy hospitals where hardly any reparative work is done.

Nurses and nursing training

Nurses are registered on separate rolls according to population group. In the past, black nurses were not represented on the South African Nursing Council, an autonomous statutory body comprising nominated and elected members and responsible, *inter alia*, for registering nurses and midwives and for setting training standards. In 1978 legislation was enacted to allow black representation on the Council, but only for nurses who are South African citizens. Those deemed to be citizens of the bantustans are excluded.

All practising midwives and nurses, students and nursing assistants are legally required to become members of the South African Nursing Association, the relevant professional body. African nurses decided in 1976 that they were against forming their own separate association in spite of being urged to do so by the Nursing Association.[33] The national management of the Association remains exclusively white, being elected by the white membership. Black nurses and midwives are only indirectly involved in the Association's activities by means of 'advisory committees', one each for African, Coloured and Indian nurses, elected by members of each population group.[34]

The racial policies of the Nursing Council led to their expulsion from the International Council of Nurses, but the Nursing Association remained unmoved. A member of the Nursing Council, a Mrs. A. van Reenen, was quoted as saying, 'It is policy that there should be racial separation. My Council wholeheartedly agrees with this. We find it necessary to effect such separation in all aspects of the nursing services.'[35]

TABLE XXVI: Registered nurses, 1980.

Population group	Number
White	28,630
Coloured	4,143
Indian	931
African	21,318
Total	55,022

Source: SAIRR, 1982, p.544, citing the 1981 Annual Report of the Department of Health, Welfare and Pensions for the numbers of nurses registered with the South African Nursing Council at 31 December 1980.

There were a total of 55,022 registered nurses in South Africa at the end of 1980, of whom 28,630 (52 per cent) were white (*see Table XXVI*). Only 20 per cent of nearly 41,000 applications for nursing training received from black people in the the Transvaal in 1978 were accepted.

The maximum number of black students who could be trained at provincial hospitals in 1979 was 3,351.[36] African nurses cannot train at Groote Schuur or at the new hospital in the Cape, Tygerberg.

According to the Minister of Health, a total of 2,761 African nurses completed their training in 1980, of whom 1,359 were general nurses, 235 general and midwifery, 1,035 midwifery and 132 psychiatric. The corresponding figures for white nurses were 883 general, 405 general and midwifery, 688 midwifery, 133 psychiatric, and 34 general and psychiatric.[37]

Nurses' salaries

In recent years there has been great dissatisfaction amongst nurses, including white nurses, over salaries. Many whites have left the profession, thus aggravating the already acute shortage of nurses. As long ago as 1971 Professor Chris Barnard was quoted as saying that Coloured nurses would have to nurse white patients because white hospitals could not cope. The fact that black hospitals were equally understaffed appeared to be overlooked. Professor Barnard's remark, however, provoked Dr. L. Munnik, a member of the Provincial Executive Council in charge of Cape hospitals, to retort that 'It will never happen as long as I am a member of the Executive Council.'[38]

In 1976 the Minister of Health announced that the government was prepared to allow black nurses to look after white patients in private hospitals provided that no white nurse was available for the job, and provided equal salaries were paid (to avoid black staff being appointed as cheaper labour). Despite this a spokesman for a private nursing home in Johannesburg subsequently said that his institution was only allowed to employ black nurses if they had no contact with white patients and that such black employees were being paid only slightly more than at provincial hospitals.[39] In Natal it was decided to allow black nurses in white private hospitals but only under constant white supervision.

Black nurses trained at Baragwanath have gone into commercial employment and private nursing homes because of the poor rates of pay at provincial hospitals.[40] Private employment is less secure, however. In 1979 Coloured nursing sisters were banned from working at an exclusive white maternity home in Johannesburg, and replaced by white nurses and assistants, some of whom had less experience and lower qualifications.[41] In general blacks may not take jobs if skilled whites are looking for employment. Furthermore, not all jobs in private homes are well paid. Reports appeared in 1977, for example, of black women employed as nurse aids in old age homes for whites who were paid only R40 to R55 per month. They were not entitled to pensions, medical aid, uniforms, or travel allowance, and they doubled up as domestics, working shifts. At

93

one home a nursing assistant was paid R40 a month for a 12 hour day. She was paid in cash and not given a pay slip.[42]

Nurses of all population groups were due to receive average salary increases of 48 per cent in October 1982, but the director of the Commission for Administration said that these were not aimed at closing the wage gap. It was left up to individual employing authorities to assess each nurse and to work out the details. The Commission also announced a restructuring of salary scales, with the existing 20 levels being reduced to 11.[43]

The position in practice after the increases varied from province to province. In the Cape Province, white and Coloured nurses already earned the same before the increases, but not nursing assistants. There was salary parity between whites and Africans only from the level of matron. After the increases, the gap between white and African nursing sisters would be more than R1,000 a year. In Natal, the discrepancy between African nursing staff and those from other population groups was going to be R882 a year on average for nursing sisters, R984 for matrons and R1,728 for staff nurses.[44]

TABLE XXVII: Nurses' salaries, 1977.

Rank	African	Rand per month Coloured/ Indian	White
Nursing assistants	60 – 72	90 – 103	110 – 121
Student nurses	70 – 84	112.5 – 129	140 – 151
Staff nurses	105 – 126	145 – 166.75	187.5 – 206
Sisters	145 – 174	195 – 224.25	250 – 275
Head matrons	295 – 474	485 – 557.75	645 – 709.5

Source: RDM, 4.8.77.

Pharmacists

There is a critical shortage of pharmacies in South Africa's black townships. In 1976 there were reported to be 51 Coloured and 122 Indian pharmacists in South Africa. The Department of Health employed 54 whites and two Indians in the pharmaceutical field, but no Africans or Coloureds.[45]

In 1973 just two Africans qualified as pharmacists together with four Coloured and 21 Indian students, making a total of 27 against 282 three year-trained and 140 four year-trained white students. In the same year

94

there were only 12 registered African chemists and druggists compared with 4,693 whites.[46] Differential salary scales apply in pharmacy as in the other professions. (*The salary scales in 1977 are indicated in Table XXVIII.*)

TABLE XXVIII: Salary scales for pharmacists, 1977.

Rank	White	Rand per annum Coloured/ Indian	African
Chief pharmacist	9,900 – 11,700	8,100 – 9,640	6,060 – 6,300
Senior pharmacist	7,740 – 9,540	6,060 – 6,300	4,740 – 7,380
Pharmacist	5,340 – 6,300	4,340 – 5,100	3,450 – 4,020
Trainee pharmacist	4,020 (fixed)	3,130 (fixed)	male: 2,100* (fixed) female: 1,980 (fixed)

* For Africans there is further discrimination in salaries on grounds of sex.

Source: Debates, 4.2.77.

Professional bodies

Medical practitioners and medical services in South Africa fall under the statutory control of the South African Medical and Dental Council. This is an autonomous body comprising members elected by the profession itself, government nominees, and others appointed by professional councils, universities and the provinces.

The Medical Association of South Africa (MASA) is a professional association of doctors with a membership of between 9 and 10,000, or around 80 per cent of all actively practising doctors.[47]

Government intervention in the affairs of the South African Medical and Dental Council increased following the introduction of new legislation in 1974. This reduced the total membership, cutting down on the numbers of members elected by doctors and dentists themselves, and the number appointed by the universities. The first appointment of a black doctor to the Council was made in 1973.[48]

Prior to 1974, the South African Medical Association, through its official organ, the *South African Medical Journal*, had a monopoly on advertising medical and dental posts in South Africa. The government took action, however, after MASA refused to accept advertisements for the *Journal* if they made reference to lower rates of pay for blacks. This was basically a cosmetic measure as blacks were barred from posts in white hospitals in any case and the advertisers only had to delete references to race and salary in the job description. Nevertheless, the *Journal* was stripped of its status as sole advertising medium for vacancies and now all state professional medical posts can be advertised in the press.[49]

During 1982 an alternative association for registered doctors and dentists from all population groups was formed in South Africa — the National Medical and Dental Association, NAMDA. It reportedly arose out of dissatisfaction among many doctors that their views were not being adequately represented by MASA, and that the latter was too closely aligned with the apartheid state. Doctors and dentists joining NAMDA were nevertheless allowed to retain their membership of MASA. A spokesman for NAMDA, Professor Jerry Coovadia, explained that a pressure group was needed to work for democratic changes in the health services and in health education. 'An alternative medical association can take up issues such as cholera and provide a public account of the causes of ill health . . . We can present to the outside world a true image of the prevailing problems in health in South Africa,' he said.[50] A member of NAMDA's new executive said that dissatisfaction with MASA had come to the fore following the public outcry over the death in detention of Steve Biko, the black consciousness leader. NAMDA felt that MASA's response to the whole question of the health and welfare of detainees under security legislation had been inadequate, he said.[51] By March 1983 branches of NAMDA had been formed in Natal, the Cape and the Transvaal.[52]

9. Doctors and the State

The relationship between doctors and the State in South Africa was highlighted by the Biko case.

Steve Biko, leader of the black consciousness movement, died while in police custody in September 1977, three weeks after he was arrested. A post mortem revealed massive brain damage and haemorrhage.

Biko was not the first political prisoner to die while in police custody, nor would he be the last, but the case provoked an international outcry partly because of glaring medical negligence on the part of the doctors who had been called in to examine him. The doctors, Dr. Ivor Lang and Dr. Benjamin Tucker, and a consultant physician, Dr. Colin Hersch, had ignored objective clinical signs of brain damage when examining Biko. Instead of ordering immediate hospitalization and surgery, they had allowed him to be transferred to a prison hospital in Pretoria, 740 miles away from Port Elizabeth where he was being held. The police had apparently suggested that Biko, being a medical student, might be malingering, and the doctors did not contradict them. One of the doctors admitted later at the inquest that 'he didn't know that in this particular situation one could override the decisions made by a responsible police officer.'[1] At the inquest the doctors admitted clinical errors, falsification of reports, and Dr. Lang admitted that he wrote out a highly incorrect medical certificate at the request of Colonel Goosen of the Security Police.

After the inquest, which took almost a year to complete and at the end found that no specific person could be blamed for Biko's death, the case was submitted to the South African Medical and Dental Council for further investigation. However, the Council decided, *in camera*, to postpone its enquiry after the State Attorney had allegedly threatened to take legal action to prevent the Council obtaining an explanation from the doctors.[2]

After almost three years of procrastination the South African Medical and Dental Council found the doctors not guilty of unprofessional conduct. They were supported in this by the Medical Association of South Africa (MASA). In spite of protests inside South Africa and abroad no further action was taken against the doctors concerned. MASA at the outset endorsed the Council's findings, stating that 'on the evidence available, MASA's Executive Committee felt that the doctors who treated Mr.

Biko had exercised reasonable skill and care and were not guilty of negligence, while no proof of improper or disgraceful conduct had been submitted'.[3] MASA reached this conclusion despite being a signatory to the 1975 Tokyo Declaration of the World Medical Association which stipulated the proper conduct of doctors towards political prisoners and detainees. (*See extract from the Tokyo Declaration adopted by the 29th World Medical Assembly of the WMA in October 1975, below.*)

Thus the Medical Association of South Africa, while adopting a stance of concern, actually did nothing apart from requesting that the Council give urgent attention to questions the answers to which were already obvious.

In August 1977 Hoosen Haffejee, a dentist aged 26 from Durban, was found dead in his cell 24 hours after being arrested under suspicion of 'terrorism'. Death was supposed to have been due to suicide by hanging.

At the inquest bruises were found all over his body and these were, according to medical evidence, inflicted pre-mortem. There was also evidence of head injuries. Professor Isadore Gordon, State Pathologist (and incidentally former Dean of Natal Medical School) said in giving evidence that the bruises were 'hard to explain'. He did admit, however, that the bruises could have been inflicted by a booted foot, the head injury also being the result of a blow. Other abrasions were described as possibly being inflicted by 'a special pair of pliers'.[4] In the face of this kind of evidence the court still returned a verdict of suicide.

Subsequent to the deaths of Biko and Haffejee there have been more deaths in detention, including that of Dr. Neil Aggett in February 1982, a case in which torture was again alleged. However, as long as no doctors are involved as was the case with Biko, the medical profession in South Africa apparently prefers to maintain a deafening silence on these issues. By the end of 1983 there had been 58 known deaths in detention in South Africa.

There are no legislative guidelines for the medical treatment of detainees, but the Department of Health has listed the doctor's obligations when treating a patient in police custody. These state that a doctor should have access to his or her patient at all times. The Prisons Act, however, makes it clear that a prison doctor can be legally overruled by a non-medical police or prison official. The Internal Security Act (which replaces the Terrorism Act) precludes a detainee from having access to a legal adviser without official permission, and this can effectively prevent the detainee from seeking judicial intervention to enforce any rights he/she may have to medical treatment.[5]

The acquiescent attitude of members of the medical profession also became apparent during the uprisings in Soweto and elsewhere in South Africa in 1976 and early 1977. There were several reports of youths, average age 12, who had been totally or partially blinded through gunshot injuries to the eyes caused by birdshot fired by the police. Hospital authorities at Baragwanath Eye Hospital refused to disclose how many children suffered such injuries.

In January 1977 the Medical Association of South Africa instructed the Ophthalmological Society to investigate the incidence of eye injuries in these cases. A report was submitted to the Medical Association which stated that it would be passed to the government and would not be made public. Speaking in the House of Assembly Helen Suzman of the Progressive Reform Party accused the medical profession of being party 'to a conspiracy of silence . . . to its eternal shame.' She revealed figures showing that 30 people in the Cape suffered eye injuries as a result of birdshot; there were no figures for the Transvaal. Of the 30, 19 suffered total blindness or severe loss of vision. Suzman expressed shock that MASA did not report its findings to the Cillie Commission which had been appointed to investigate the unrest in the country. In reply, Dr. C. Viljoen, General Secretary of MASA, said that the Association 'did not have substantiated evidence of a single injury caused by birdshot.'[6]

Relationship with world medical bodies

In spite of MASA's poor record in exposing the injustices in South African society, South Africa was re-admitted to the World Medical Association (WMA) in 1981. It had resigned in 1975 after its delegation had been refused visas by the Japanese government to attend the Tokyo assembly of the World Medical Association. The Secretary General of the WMA, Dr. Andre Wynan, claimed in 1981 that the quality of medicine in South Africa was among the best in the world and said that MASA's re-admission to the WMA was a mere formality.[7]

The Transkei Medical Association in the Transkei bantustan applied for and secured admission to the WMA at the same time. The World Medical Association amended its constitution following its assembly in Tokyo to allow proportional voting of its members, thus ensuring that the American, West German and Japanese medical associations held a voting majority. This enabled the WMA to pass a resolution that congresses be held only in those countries which could not refuse visas to any of its delegates. Eleven Third World countries, and recently Britain, have since withdrawn their membership of the WMA in protest at its attitude towards South Africa, and the World Health Organisation has withdrawn its recognition of the WMA.

Extract from the Tokyo Declaration adopted by the 29th World Medical Assembly of the World Medical Association (WMA) in October 1975

(The Medical Association of South Africa [MASA] is a signatory of this Declaration.)

'The doctor shall not countenance, condone or participate in the practice of torture or other forms of cruel, inhuman or degrading procedures whatever the offence of which the victim of such procedures is suspected, accused or guilty, and whatever the victim's beliefs or motives, and in situations including armed conflict and civil strife.

'A doctor must have complete clinical independence in deciding upon the care of a person for whom he or she is medically responsible.

'The doctor shall in all circumstances be bound to alleviate the distress of his fellow men and no motive — whether personal, collective or political — shall prevail against this higher purpose.'

10. Conclusion

Health in South Africa is inseparable from the economic, political and social structure of the apartheid state. The question that arises for those engaged in health work in South Africa is whether the political situation has become so difficult that effective work is impossible. Malnutrition, which is a direct result of the government's policies, is a classic example of this dilemma. South African paediatricians have developed an expertise in the understanding and treatment of malnutrition and its complications, but this has done nothing to change the system which gives rise to the disease. After expert treatment children are returned to an environment where they will in all probability relapse and where at least half will die before their fifth birthday. It has been said that South Africa does not have a health service, but a disease service, and this sums up the position very accurately.

Health workers are in a dilemma. There is a growing realisation that providing good health services does not depend so much on the skill of doctors and other health personnel but rather on the prevailing political, social and economic conditions. The evidence in this book leads to the conclusion that the present apartheid system needs to be completely dismantled if the health of all South Africans is to improve. In its place must come a new social order to provide full employment, free and compulsory education, decent housing and recreational facilities, decent living wages and a free and readily available health service to all the people of South Africa.

Abbreviations and References

CH   *Cape Herald*, Cape Town.
CT   *Cape Times*, Cape Town.
Cit   *The Citizen*, Johannesburg.
DD   *Daily Dispatch*, East London.
Debates   *House of Assembly Debates (Hansard)*, Cape Town/Pretoria.
DN   *Daily News*, Durban.
FM   *Financial Mail*, Johannesburg.
FOCUS   *Focus on Political Repression in Southern Africa*, bimonthly news bulletin of IDAF.
GG   *Government Gazette*, Pretoria.
GN   *The Guardian*, London.
NM   *Natal Mercury*, Durban.
NW   *Natal Witness*, Pietermaritzburg.
Post   *Post*, Johannesburg.
RDM   *Rand Daily Mail*, Johannesburg.
S   *Sowetan*, Johannesburg.
SAIRR   *Survey of Race Relations in South Africa*, South African Institute of Race Relations, Johannesburg (published annually).
SALB   *South African Labour Bulletin*.
SALDRU   *Southern African Labour and Development Research Unit*.
SAMJ   *South African Medical Journal*.
SAMST   South African Medical Scholarship Trust.
S.Exp   *Sunday Express*, Johannesburg.
ST   *Sunday Times*, Johannesburg.
Star   *Star*, Johannesburg.
S. Tribune *Sunday Tribune*, Durban.
T   *The Times*, London.
Tel   *Daily Telegraph*, London.
World   *World*, Johannesburg,

1. Introduction — Some Statistics

1. *Official Year Book of the Republic of South Africa*, 1983.
2. H. C. J. van Rensburg & A. Mans, *Profile of Disease and Health Care in South Africa*, Academica, Pretoria/Cape Town/Johannesburg, 1982, p.23; *Official Year Book, op. cit.*
3. *CT*, 26.5.83.
4. L. G. Wells, *Health, healing and society*, Ravan Press, Johannesburg, 1974, p.3.
5. *Official Year Book, op. cit.*
6. *Official Year Book of the RSA*, 1980/81.
7. David Bourne & Bruce Dick, 'Mortality in South Africa — 1924-1974', in *Perspectives on the Health System*, ed. Gill Westcott & Francis Wilson, SALDRU/SAMST, Ravan Press, Johannesburg, 1979.
8. *Official Year Book of the RSA*, 1983.
9. *RDM*, 24.8.82.
10. H. C. Seftel, Professor of African Diseases, University of the Witwatersrand, *Medicine and society in South Africa — Some plain speaking*, inaugural lecture, University of the Witwatersrand, 14.8.73.
11. *Debates*, 20.3.79, table of notifiable diseases.

12. L. G. Wells, *op. cit.*, p.2.
13. M. D. McGrath, 'Health expenditure in South Africa', in *Perspectives on the Health System*, op. cit.
14. H. C. Seftel, 'A sick society', *FM*, 2.3.79.
15. *RDM*, 13.10.80.
16. *SAMJ*, Vol. 53, 1978, p.503.
17. Jonathan Brodie, 'The ethical drug manufacturing industry in South Africa', in *Hunger, Work and Health*, ed. Gill Westcott & Francis Wilson, SALDRU/SAMST, Ravan Press, Johannesburg, 1980.
18. *Debates*, 28.2.77, col. 2377.
19. *Tel*, 11.11.81.
20. Medical Students Council *et. al.*, *Training and testing of medical students — a diagnostic appraisal*, SALDRU/SAMST conference, September 1978, *op. cit.*
21. *ibid.*
22. *Report XI from South Africa*, South African Embassy, London, 1975, p.9.
23. *BBC Television*, 12.12.74.

2. The Bantustans, Migrant Labour and Poverty

1. Colin Bundy, in *African Affairs* Vol. 71 No. 285, October 1975.
2. Quoted in Aninka Claassens, 'An assessment of self-help projects in a district of Transkei', in *Hunger, Work and Health*, ed. Gill Westcott & Francis Wilson, SALDRU/SAMST, Ravan Press, Johannesburg, 1980.
3. *Nutrition and the Bantu*, pamphlet published by the SA Department of Information, December 1971.
4. *SAIRR*, 1982, pp. 45, 372.
5. *ibid.*, p.43; *Official Year Book of the Republic of South Africa*, 1980/81.
6. *SAIRR*, 1982, p.45.
7. *ibid.*, p.409.
8. *ibid.*, p.413.
9. *ibid.*, pp. 409, 45.
10. *Apartheid — The Facts*, IDAF, London, 1983, p.40.
11. Quoted in David Davis, *African Workers and Apartheid*, IDAF, London, 1978, p.5.
12. *Apartheid — The Facts, op. cit.*, p.44.
13. *Debates*, 24.6.68.
14. *Apartheid — The Facts, op. cit.*, p.23.
15. H. C. J. van Rensburg & A. Mans, *Profile of Disease and Health Care in South Africa*, Academica, Pretoria/Cape Town/Johannesburg, 1982, p.44, citing official figures published by the 1976 Theron Commission.
16. *SAIRR*, 1982, p.412; *Africa Guide 1982*, ed. Enver Carim, World of Information, 1982.
17. *SAIRR*, 1982, p.70. The figures exclude Transkei, Bophuthatswana and Venda.
18. Peter Randall (ed), *Power, Privilege and Poverty* (Report of the Economics Commission of SPRO-CAS), SPRO-CAS, Johannesburg, 1972.

19. *SAIRR*, 1978, p.207.
20. *Apartheid — The Facts, op. cit.*, p.46.
21. SPRO-CAS, *op. cit.*, and see Table III.
22. *SAIRR*, 1982, p.64, and see Table III.
23. *FM*, 19.11.76.
24. *X-Ray*, July-August 1976.
25. *SAIRR*, 1982, p.67.
26. *ibid*, p.67.
27. *ibid*, pp. 67-8.
28. H. C. J. van Rensburg & A. Mans, *op. cit.*, p.51.
29. *FM*, 11.1.80.
30. C. E. W. Simkins, 'Measuring and predicting unemployment in South Africa', in *Structural Unemployment in South Africa*, Natal University Press, 1978.
31. *South African Unemployment: A Black Picture*, ed. C. E. W. Simkins & C. Desmond, University of Natal, 1978.
32. *SAIRR*, 1982, p.71.
33. *ibid*, p.73.
34. *ibid*, pp. 73-4.

3. Malnutrition and Infant Mortality

1. Trudy Thomas, 'The effectiveness of alternative methods of managing malnutrition', in *Hunger, Work and Health*, ed. Gill Westcott & Francis Wilson, SALDRU/SAMST, Ravan Press, Johannesburg, 1980.
2. Liz Clarke, 'The need for a community development approach to combating malnutrition,' in *Hunger, Work and Health, op. cit.*
3. *SAMJ*, Vol. 47, 1973, p.702.
4. H. C. J. van Rensburg & A. Mans, *Profile of Disease and Health Care in South Africa*, Academica, Pretoria/Cape Town/Johannesburg, 1982, p.171.
5. *ibid*.
6. *Debates*, 2.5.80.
7. *Report of the Ciskei Commission (Quail Report)*, 1980, p. 30, cited in H. C. J. van Rensburg & A. Mans, *op. cit.*, p.172.
8. *RDM*, 13.12.80.
9. *Star*, 24.8.80.
10. *RDM*, 14.5.80.
11. *NW*, 13.9.79.
12. *CH*, 23.4.83.
13. *S*, 14.4.83.
14. *DN*, 2.2.83.
15. *SAMJ*, Vol. 55, p. 796, 12.5.79.
16. *Official Year Book of the Republic of South Africa*, 1980/81, and see Chapter 1.
17. *Official Year Book of the RSA*, 1983.
18. *World*, 7.11.76.
19. *Star*, 20.2.71.
20. *RDM*, 13.12.80.
21. J. V. O. Reid, 'Malnutrition', paper prepared for the National Union of South African Students (NUSAS), published by SAIRR, August 1971.
22. *Star*, 20.12.80.
23. *RDM*, 21.7.80.
24. Reid, *op. cit.*
25. H. C. Seftel, *Medicine and society in South Africa — Some plain speaking*, inaugural lecture, University of the Witwatersrand, 14.8.73.
26. *RDM*, 8.6.74.
27. *SA Outlook*, 1976.
28. *Star*, 12.6.76.
29. *Star*, 5.8.82.

30. *RDM*, 26.6.81.
31. *SAMJ*, Vol. 39, 1965 & 22.7.67.

4. Infectious Diseases

1. *DD*, 16.9.80; *Star*, 3.8.82.
2. *Star*, 28.4.81, 3.8.82; *SAIRR*, 1982, p.527.
3. *DD*, 16.9.80.
4. *SAIRR*, 1982, p.527.
5. *The Lancet*, 11.4.80.
6. *SAIRR*, 1982, p.526.
7. H. C. J. van Rensburg & A. Mans, *Profile of Disease and Health Care in South Africa*, Academica, Pretoria/Cape Town/Johannesburg, 1982, p.149.
8. *CT*, 10.5.78.
9. *SAIRR*, 1982, p.528.
10. *CT*, 10.5.78.
11. *Debates*, 6.4.79.
12. *Star*, 5.8.82.
13. *S. Tribune*, 1.10.78.
14. *S. Exp.*, 4.10.81.
15. *Star*, 22.7.82; and see Table X.
16. *SAIRR*, 1981, p.401.
17. *CT*, 1.7.82.
18. *ibid*.
19. *T.*, 13.3.81.
20. *RDM*, 2.12.81.
21. *CT*, 1.7.82.
22. *Debates*, 14.2.83; *RDM*, 15.2.83.
23. *CT*, 2.4.82; cited in *SAIRR*, 1982, p.530.
24. *DN*, 24.3.83.
25. *SAMJ*, 14.12.74, Vol. 48, p.2557.
26. *SAIRR*, 1982, p.530.
27. *S*, 15.4.83; *RDM*, 12.5.83.
28. H. C. J. van Rensburg & A. Mans, *op. cit.*, p.160.
29. *RDM*, 14.7.82.
30. Robert Scott, *Health services in Graaf Reinet*, paper presented to SALDRU/SAMST conference on the economics of health care in southern Africa, University of Cape Town, September 1978.
31. *Implications of apartheid on health and health services in South Africa*, by a group of black doctors in South Africa, UN Centre against Apartheid, *Notes and Documents*, No. 18/77, June 1977.
32. *CT*, 8.9.82.
33. *ibid*.
34. *SASPU National*, October 1981.
35. *SAIRR*, 1982, pp. 531-2; and see Table IX.
36. *ibid*, pp. 532-3.
37. *SAIRR*, 1982, p.533.
38. *Debates*, 10.3.83.
39. *SAIRR*, 1982, p.533.
40. *CH*, 26.2.83.

5. Occupational Health

1. 'Economics of health care', *Social Dynamics*, University of Cape Town, Vol. 4 No. 2, 1978, p.138.
2. *SAIRR*, 1982, p.142; *Debates*, 11.4.83.
3. *SAIRR, ibid*.
4. *Commission of Enquiry into Occupational Health*, (Erasmus Commission), 1976, analysed in *SALB*, Vol. 4, Nos. 9 & 10, March 1979.
5. *ibid*.
6. *ibid*.
7. *NM*, 24.7.81.

8. Erasmus Commission/*SALB, op. cit.*
9. *ibid.*
10. *ibid.*
11. *RDM,* 18.11.81; *CT,* 18/27.11.81; *ST,* 6.12.81.
12. *ST,* 6.12.81; *CT,* 27.11.81.
13. *RDM/CT,* 18.11.81.
14. *ST,* 5.9.82.
15. *CT,* 17.12.82.
16. *FM,* 15.4.81.
17. *S.Exp.* 23.8.81.
18. *ST,* 5.9.82.
19. *Multinational Monitor,* March 1982; *New Statesman,* 11.12.81.
20. Erasmus Commission/*SALB, op. cit.*
21. *CT,* 16.7.76; *RDM,* 25.6.76.
22. *RDM,* 28.4.82.
23. *RDM,* 10.12.81.
24. *FM,* 18.8.78.
25. A. Pokrovsky, *African labour in the mines of South Africa,* UN Centre against Apartheid, Notes and Documents No. 20/73, November 1973.
26. Act No. 78 of 1973, *GG,* 8976, 6.3.73.
27. *Critical Health,* No. 8, September 1982.
28. *RDM,* 10.4.74, 6/8.5.74.
29. *SAMJ,* 14.12.74.
30. *S,* 3.6.82.
31. *Star,* 2.4.78.

6. Mental Health

1. F. de Villiers, *ST,* 27.4.78.
2. Richard West, *Spectator,* 9.6.79.
3. *ibid.*
4. *Debates,* 14.12.77.
5. *SAIRR,* 1981, p.402.
6. *CT,* 1.2.80, cited in *'If we gave them shoes . . . they would kick their fellow patients' — The case for South Africa's expulsion from international psychiatry,* Anti-Apartheid Movement, London, July 1983.
7. *CT,* 1.2.80; cited in Anti-Apartheid Movement, *op. cit.*
8. *Debates,* 14.12.77.
9. 'Report of the Committee to visit South Africa — Official Action of the American Psychiatric Association', *American Journal of Psychiatry,* 136:11, November 1979.
10. *Apartheid and Mental Health Care,* Report by the World Health Organisation, UN Centre against Apartheid, *Notes and Documents,* 11/77, April 1977.
11. APA Report, *op. cit.*
12. *CT,* 25.5.76.
13. APA Report, *op. cit.*
14. *ibid.*
15. *ibid.*
16. *ibid.*
17. *Star,* 21.2.76.
18. *RDM,* 27.6.77.
19. APA Report, *op. cit.*
20. Report by the World Health Organisation, *op. cit.*
21. *RDM,* 2.5.80.
22. *SAIRR,* 1980, p.562.
23. *SAIRR,* 1981, p.402, 1982, p.538.
24. *ibid.*
25. *RDM,* 2.8.83.
26. *SAIRR,* 1982, p.538.

27. Dr. P. J. Henning, 'Mental health facilities', in *Race Relations News,* Vol. 38, 1976.
28. *ibid.*
29. *RDM* 11.1.82.
30. Report of the World Health Organisation, *op. cit.*
31. Director General of the World Health Organisation, *Health implications of apartheid in South Africa,* UN Notes and Documents, March 1975; *Clinical Medicine in Africans in Southern Africa,* ed. G. D. Campbell, Y. K. Seedat, & G. Daynes (Churchill Livingstone, 1973).
32. *Clinical Medicine, op. cit.*
33. *Apartheid and Mental Health Care, op. cit.*
34. *FM,* 11.5.69.
35. *DD,* 18.7.80.
36. APA Report, *op. cit.*
37. *SAIRR,* 1981, pp. 402-3.
38. Anti-Apartheid Movement, July 1983, *op. cit.*
39. *CT,* 14.8.82; *S,* 28.10.82.
40. *ibid.*
41. *RDM,* 16.11.76.
42. *W,* 15.8.77.
43. *ibid.*
44. H. C. J. van Rensburg & A. Mans, *Profile of Disease and Health Care in South Africa,* Academica, Pretoria/Cape Town/Johannesburg, 1982, pp. 78-9.
45. *RDM,* 15.7.77.
46. W. Louw, *Alcoholism and liquor abuse in the Western Cape,* paper presented to SALDRU/SAMST conference on the economics of health care in southern Africa, University of Cape Town, September 1978.
47. *ibid.*
48. *CT,* 26.1.79.
49. *Post,* 10.8.78.
50. *FM,* 24.3.78.
51. *RDM,* 5.6.78.
52. *DN,* 2.7.82.
53. Report by the World Health Organisation, *op. cit.*

7. Health Services

1. L. G. Wells, *Health, healing and society,* Ravan Press, Johannesburg, 1974.
2. 'Soweto — A survey', *FM supplement,* 25.3.83; *RDM,* 24.5.76.
3. *South African Review I, Same Foundations, New Facade?* ed. & compiled by South African Research Services, Ravan Press, Johannesburg, 1983.
4. *RDM,* 2.8.83.
5. *ST,* 7.8.77.
6. *Star,* 15.10.82; *S,* 28.1.83.
7. *Star, ibid.*
8. *S,* 28.1.83.
9. *S,* 11.10.82.
10. *S,* 22.2.83.
11. *S,* 19.10.82.
12. *CT,* 26.6.76.
13. *CT,* 7.12.82.
14. *CT,* 11.8.82, 28.1.83.
15. *FM,* 1.8.78.
16. *S,* 5.10.82.
17. *DD,* 2.6.78.
18. *SAIRR,* 1982, p.539, quoting Dr. Anthony Zwi, *'Homeland' Tragedy: Function and Farce,* Development Studies Group/South African Research Services, August 1982.

104

19. *Debates*, 24.2.76.
20. *SAIRR*, 1982, p.541.
21. *ibid.*
22. SALDRU/SAMST conference on the economics of health care in Southern Africa, University of Cape Town, September 1978.
23. *S*, 1.10.82.
24. *S*, 22.2.83.
25. *SAIRR*, 1982, p.536.
26. *RDM*, 11.3.77; *South African Review I, op. cit.*
27. *Debates*, 24.2.76.
28. *RDM*, 2.11.82.
29. *ST*, 6.2.83.
30. *GN/Tel*, 15.7.83.
31. *Tel*, 15.7.83.
32. *S.Exp*, 15.8.82.
33. *S*, 9.2.83.
34. *Post*, 26.4.79.
35. *ST*, 31.10.82.
36. *Regulations for the control of blood transfusion services, GG Extraordinary, IV,* 385 Regulation Gazette No. 146, Second schedule, A 23(2)(b), p.36.
37. *Genetically determined hazards of blood transfusion within and between races,* SAMJ, 13.1.73, Vol. 47, p.56.
38. *RDM.,* 9.1.84; *S. Tribune,* 8.1.84.
39. *GN.,* 26.8.82; *ST,* 29.8.82.
40. *S,* 20.7.82.
41. H. C. J. van Rensburg & A. Mans, *Profile of Disease and Health Care in South Africa,* Academica, Pretoria/Cape Town/Johannesburg, 1982, p.266.
42. *ibid,* p.269.
43. *FM,* 24.3.78.
44. *RDM,* 2.11.82.
45. *FM,* 21.1.83.
46. *SAIRR,* 1982, p.551.
47. *ibid.*
48. *ibid.*
49. *Debates,* 19.6.76.
50. *DN,* 20.9.82.
51. *SAIRR,* 1982, p.552.
52. *RDM,* 14.3.77.
53. *SAIRR,* 1982, p.553.
54. *ST,* 14.11.82.
55. *CT,* 31.3.83.
56. *Post,* 23.12.79.
57. *SAIRR,* 1982, p.550.
58. *ibid.*
59. *ibid,* p.551.
60. *RDM,* 1.3.77.
61. *SAIRR,* 1982, pp. 550-1.
62. *ibid,* p.551.
63. *W,* 10.8.77.
64. *SAIRR,* 1982, p.554.
65. *ibid.*
66. *ibid.*
67. *Star,* 26.6.82, 22.8.83; *S. Exp,* 5.9.82.
68. *DN,* 16.11.82.
69. *DN,* 1.12.82.
70. *S.Exp,* 6.6.82.
71. *DN,* 2.3.83.
72. *DN,* 19.7.83.
73. *Star,* 26.9.82.

8. Health Workers

1. *SAIRR*, 1982, p.542.
2. H. C. J. van Rensburg & A. Mans, *Profile of Disease and Health Care in South Africa,* Academica, Pretoria/Cape Town/Johannesburg, 1982, p.215, citing SA Dept. of Information publication of 1977.
3. *ibid,* pp. 211, 216.
4. Ralph Kirsch, 'Health needs in Southern Africa,' in *Perspectives on the Health System,* ed. Gill Westcott & Francis Wilson, SALDRU/SAMST, Ravan Press, Johannesburg, 1979.
5. H. C. J. van Rensburg & A. Mans, *op. cit.,* p.211.
6. *ibid,* p.221.
7. Tim Wilson, 'The need for health professionals in South Africa', in *Hunger, Work and Health,* ed. Gill Westcott & Francis Wilson, SALDRU/SAMST, Ravan Press, Johannesburg, 1980.
8. *SAIRR*, 1982, p.542.
9. *RDM,* 18.11.69.
10. *SAIRR*, 1982, p.546.
11. *FM,* 12.11.82.
12. Prof. P. V. Tobias, University of Witwatersrand Medical School, *Apartheid and Medical Education,* address given to the Social Action Group of the Medical Students Council, 7.6.1979.
13. *CT,* 27.4.76.
14. Prof. P. V. Tobias, *op. cit.*
15. Dr. H. F. Verwoerd, Minister of Native Affairs, speaking in the Senate, 7.6.54.
16. I. B. Tabata, *Education for Barbarism,* Durban, 1959.
17. *SAIRR*, 1982, pp. 463-5.
18. *Debates*, 23.2.83, 30.3.82.
19. *Star*, 29.9.74.
20. *CT*, 1.4.74.
21. *RDM*, 5.2.76; *Star*, 21.2.76.
22. *RDM*, 6.5.77.
23. Dr. Gale, writing in the *Proceedings of the Medical Association for the Prevention of War,* Vol. 2. 1974, Parts 9 & 10.
24. *T*, 21.8.78.
25. *RDM*, 1.12.77.
26. *Star*, 16.6.69.
27. *Debates*, 8.2.72.
28. *RDM*, 11.7.70, 7/15.8.70; *Debates*, 24.7.70.
29. *SAIRR*, 1982, p.544.
30. *RDM*, 13.10.80.
31. *RDM*, 20.11.68.
32. *SAIRR*, 1980, p.574.
33. *RDM*, 16.2.76.
34. H. C. J. van Rensburg & S. A. Mans, *op. cit.,* p.235.
35. *Report of the Select Committee on the Subject of the Nursing Amendment Bill,* House of Assembly, 1955, and *Debates,* 1957.
36. *Star*, 15.2.79.
37. *SAIRR*, 1981, p.408.
38. *CT*, 13.3.71.
39. *RDM*, 4.8.77.
40. *FM*, 24.11.78.
41. *GN*, 19.5.79.
42. *W*, 13.9.77.
43. *SAIRR*, 1982, p.545.
44. *ibid.*
45. *Debates*, 7.5.76.
46. *Debates*, 20.8.73.
47. H. C. J. van Rensburg & A. Mans, *op. cit.,* p.212.
48. *RDM*, 21.12.73.
49. *CT*, 30.5.74.

50. *DD*, 17.12.82.
51. *DN*, 10.12.82.
52. *DD*, 24.3.83.

9. Doctors and the State

1. Hilda Bernstein, *No. 46 – Steve Biko*, IDAF, London, 1978.
2. *RDM*, 30.10.78.
3. Quoted in *Memorandum to the World Medical Association*, signed by 15 health organisations in South Africa and reproduced by the Anti-Apartheid Movement Health Committee, London, 1981.
4. *FOCUS*, 16. p.12.
5. *Star*, 30.8.81.
6. *SAIRR*, 1977, pp.111-2.
7. *Cit/RDM*, 9.7.81.

106

Index

.

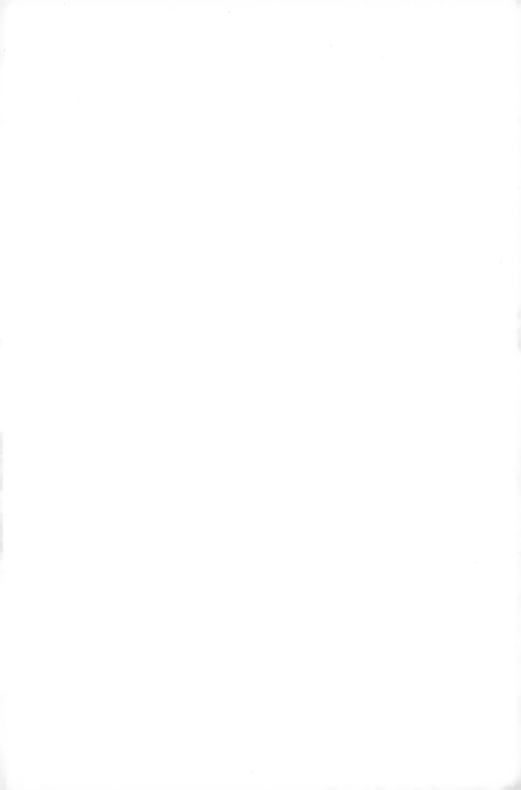

Printed in England by A G Bishop & Sons Ltd, Orpington, Kent.